HEALING WITH VAGUS NERVE EXERCISES

ACTIVATE THE BODY'S SUPERPOWER TO REGULATE YOUR NERVOUS SYSTEM - DAILY ROUTINES TO MANAGE ANXIETY, PAIN, INSOMNIA, FATIGUE, GUT HEALTH AND INFLAMMATION

J.C MYLES

Copyright © 2025 by J.C MYLES

All rights reserved.

No portion of this book may be reproduced in any form without written permission from the publisher or author, except as permitted by U.S. copyright law.

This publication is designed to provide accurate and authoritative information in regard to the subject matter covered. It is sold with the understanding that neither the author nor the publisher is engaged in rendering legal, investment, accounting or other professional services.

While the publisher and author have used their best efforts in preparing this book, they make no representations or warranties with respect to the accuracy or completeness of the contents of this book and specifically disclaim any implied warranties of merchantability or fitness for a particular purpose.

No warranty may be created or extended by sales representatives or written sales materials. The advice and strategies contained herein may not be suitable for your situation. You should consult with a professional when appropriate.

Neither the publisher nor the author shall be liable for any loss of profit or any other commercial damages, including but not limited to special, incidental, consequential, personal, or other damages.

First edition 2025

CONTENTS

Introduction	v
1. Understanding The Vagus Nerve	1
2. Scientific Backing and Evidence	9
3. Mental Health Healing Exercises	19
4. Physical Health Healing Exercises	31
5. PTSD and Trauma Recovery Exercises	45
6. Holistic Weight Loss Exercises	57
7. Yoga and Physical Exercises	67
8. Deep Sleep Strategies	81
9. Cold Exposure Techniques	91
10. Diet and Lifestyle Changes	101
11. Real-Life Case Studies	111
12. Integrating Vagus Nerve Exercises into Daily Life	121
Conclusion	129
References	131

INTRODUCTION

In a small town in Ohio, a man named John struggled with relentless digestive issues and chronic stress that seemed to rule his life. Traditional remedies failed him, leaving him frustrated and hopeless. One day, a friend introduced him to the concept of the vagus nerve and its exercises. Skeptical yet desperate, John began practicing these simple exercises daily. Within weeks, he noticed significant improvements in his digestion and a remarkable reduction in stress. John's story highlights the transformative potential of understanding and stimulating the vagus nerve.

Many have experienced profound healing through these exercises, and this book aims to guide you on a similar journey. I have dedicated my life to helping people overcome challenges like anxiety, pain, stress, trauma, depression, gut health issues, and inflammation. My passion for this work stems from witnessing the transformative power of simple, effective practices. I wrote this book to share reputable, easy-to-follow guidance anyone can incorporate into their daily life. I aim to offer tools that promote relaxation, homeostasis, and overall well-being.

INTRODUCTION

The purpose of this book is clear: to educate you on the importance of the vagus nerve and provide practical exercises to help you heal. We will focus on actionable daily practices that can alleviate various conditions. This book is designed to be a practical guide, offering you steps to improve your mental and physical health.

So, what is the vagus nerve? It is a crucial part of your body's parasympathetic nervous system. It extends from your brainstem to your abdomen, influencing your heart, lungs, and digestive tract. The vagus nerve regulates stress, inflammation, and emotional well-being. When stimulated, it promotes relaxation and helps maintain balance in your body and mind.

The polyvagal theory, developed by Dr. Stephen Porges, provides the scientific foundation for understanding the vagus nerve's role in health. This theory explores how the vagus nerve impacts our physiological and emotional states. It explains how activating the vagus nerve can shift our bodies from stress to calm states. This book will introduce you to the polyvagal theory and offer evidence-based exercises to stimulate your vagus nerve.

Throughout the chapters, you will find specific exercises designed to activate your vagus nerve. These practices include deep breathing, cold exposure, and mindful meditation. Real-life case studies will illustrate the positive impact of these exercises. You will also find scientific evidence supporting the benefits of vagus nerve stimulation. With practical tips, I will help you integrate these exercises into your daily routine.

This book is for anyone looking to improve their mental and physical health through natural methods. Whether you are health-conscious, struggling with specific health issues, or a professional in the health field, this book will provide you with useful knowledge and practical techniques .I encourage you to commit to trying these exercises and integrating them into your daily life. The poten-

INTRODUCTION

tial benefits are profound. By following the guidance in this book, you can significantly improve your well-being.

My research is focused on the nervous system's role in health and disease. I have studied extensively on topics related to stress, inflammation, and emotional regulation. I am committed to helping people achieve better health through holistic natural methods.

As you begin this journey, remember that small, consistent efforts can lead to significant changes. The exercises and practices in this book are designed to be simple yet effective. Dedicating a few minutes each day can activate your body's natural healing abilities and improve your emotional and nervous system regulation.

Thank you for choosing this book to explore this path to better health. Let's embark on this journey together, discovering the power of the vagus nerve and unlocking the potential for a healthier, happier life.

INTRODUCTION

BONUS

WORKBOOK & FLASHCARDS

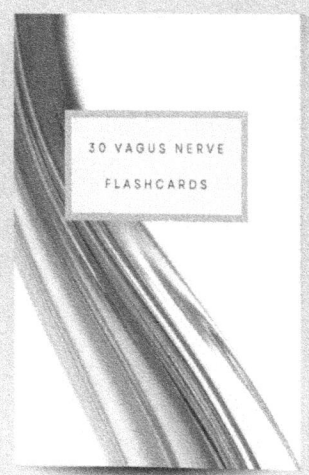 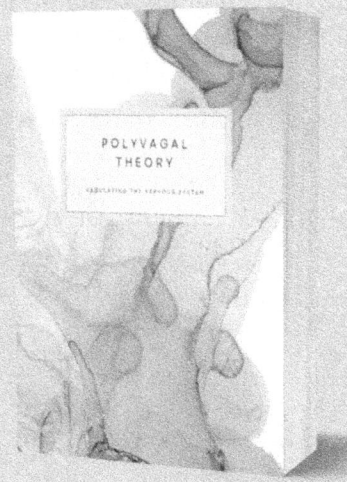

DOWNLOAD AT THE END OF THE BOOK

INTRODUCTION

At the end of chapters three to nine, you'll find a QR code linking to video classes designed to guide you through the vagus nerve exercises

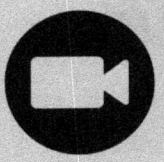

CHAPTER 1
UNDERSTANDING THE VAGUS NERVE

ANATOMY OF THE VAGUS NERVE: A CLEAR OVERVIEW

This chapter will provide you with a clear overview of the vagus nerve, its anatomy, and it's critical functions. The vagus nerve, also known as the cranial nerve X, is the longest nerve in your body. It originates in the medulla oblongata, a part of your brainstem. From there, it traverses through your neck, thorax, and abdomen, interacting with various organs along the way. This journey makes it essential for regulating numerous bodily functions. The vagus nerve exits the skull via the jugular foramen and travels within the carotid sheath alongside the carotid arteries and the internal jugular vein. As it descends, it branches out to serve various organ systems, such as the heart, lungs, and digestive tract.

One interesting quality of the vagus nerve is its dual function. It contains both afferent and efferent fibers, making it a bidirectional communicator between the brain and body. The sensory (afferent) fibers of the vagus nerve monitor the functions of various organs and send information about the state of the body back to the brain. These sensory signals include data on heart rate, digestion, and even inflammation levels.

On the other hand, the motor (efferent) fibers control muscles and glands. They send signals from the brain to the organs, instructing them to perform specific functions like slowing down heart rate or stimulating digestive processes. This dual function underscores the vagus nerve's role in maintaining homeostasis and regulating bodily functions.

The vagus nerve has a big role to play in the autonomic nervous system, specifically within the parasympathetic branch. The autonomic nervous system regulates involuntary bodily functions and is split into the sympathetic and parasympathetic divisions. The sympathetic system triggers the "fight or flight" response during stressful situations, while the parasympathetic system promotes the "rest and digest" functions. The parasympathetic system helps to calm your body after stress, reduce heart rate, stimulate digestion, and promote recovery.

Visual diagrams can significantly help you understand the vagus nerve's complex pathways and interactions. Diagrams of the vagus nerve pathways can illustrate its extensive reach from the brainstem through the neck, chest, and abdomen. These diagrams can illustrate the branches of the vagus nerve and its connections to key organs, including the heart, lungs, and digestive system. Additionally, illustrations showing nerve interactions with these organs can provide a clearer picture of how the vagus nerve influences various physiological processes. Understanding the anatomy of the vagus nerve is the first step in appreciating its role in your health.

CHAPTER 1

THE ROLE OF THE VAGUS NERVE IN THE PARASYMPATHETIC NERVOUS SYSTEM

The parasympathetic nervous system is a fundamental branch of your autonomic nervous system, which governs involuntary bodily functions. While the sympathetic nervous system gears your body up for "fight or flight" responses during stress, the parasympathetic system is responsible for your body's "rest and digest" functions that maintain balance and promote recovery. The primary function of vagal tone is to conserve energy by reducing heart rate, enhancing intestinal and glandular activity, and relaxing the sphincter muscles within the gastrointestinal tract. By fostering a state of calm and relaxation, the parasympathetic nervous system allows your body to recover from stress and maintain homeostasis.

The vagus nerve is a crucial element of the parasympathetic nervous system. It plays several roles that contribute to your overall well-being. One of its primary functions is reducing the heart rate. By sending calming signals to the heart, the vagus nerve helps lower the heart rate and promote relaxation. This is particularly important after periods of stress or physical exertion.

Additionally, the vagus nerve stimulates digestive processes, ensuring that your body can break down food and absorb nutrients. It sends a signal to the stomach and intestines to promote peristalsis, which is wave-like contractions that move food through the digestive tract. Moreover, the vagus nerve plays a big role in promoting relaxation and recovery by activating the parasympathetic response, which counteracts the stress-induced fight-or-flight response.

These functions of the vagus nerve are deeply intertwined with various physiological processes. For instance, heart rate variability (HRV) measures the variation in time between each heartbeat. Higher HRV is linked to a superior ability to adapt to stress and better cardiovascular health. The vagus nerve influences HRV by promoting a calm and steady heart rate, which can help your body respond more flexibly to stressors. Regarding digestive health, the vagus nerve stimulates gastrointestinal motility and enzyme secretion. This ensures your digestive system operates smoothly, reducing bloating, indigestion, and constipation. The vagus nerve also affects respiratory rate and depth, promoting slower, deeper breaths that enhance oxygen exchange and reduce feelings of anxiety.

Scientific evidence supports the vital role of the vagus nerve in these systems. For example, research on vagus nerve stimulation has shown significant reductions in heart rate, demonstrating its powerful effect on cardiovascular health. Studies have also highlighted the impact of vagus nerve activity on digestive health. One such study found that stimulating the vagus nerve improved gastrointestinal motility and reduced symptoms of irritable bowel syndrome (IBS). These findings underscore the importance of the vagus nerve in maintaining physiological balance and promoting overall health.

Integrating vagus nerve exercises into your daily routine can profoundly affect your well-being. Techniques such as deep breathing, mindfulness meditation, and cold exposure can stimulate the vagus nerve and activate the parasympathetic response. Regularly practicing these exercises can enhance your vagal tone, improve heart rate variability, support digestive health, and promote relaxation and recovery. The scientific evidence and real-life examples presented in this book will guide you in harnessing the power of the vagus nerve to achieve better mental and physical health.

CHAPTER 1

POLYVAGAL THEORY: SCIENTIFIC INSIGHTS AND PRACTICAL IMPLICATIONS

Dr. Stephen Porges' Polyvagal Theory offers a revolutionary perspective on how our nervous system influences behavior and health. Developed in the mid-1990s, this theory delves into the complexities of the vagus nerve, shedding light on its evolutionary role in human survival. Dr. Porges discovered that the vagus nerve is not just a simple nerve but a sophisticated system that has evolved to help mammals, including humans, respond to their environment. The theory underscores the vagus nerve's critical role in social behavior, emotional regulation, and physiological states.

Polyvagal theory identifies three distinct neural circuits that correspond to different physiological responses. The first circuit is the dorsal vagal complex, which mediates the immobilization response. This ancient system, inherited from our reptilian ancestors, activates during life-threatening situations, causing a freeze response. When this circuit is dominant, the body shuts down to conserve energy and protect itself from harm. This response can be seen in extreme stress or trauma situations, where individuals may feel numb or detached.

The second circuit involves the sympathetic nervous system, responsible for the mobilization response, commonly known as the "fight or flight" reaction. When faced with danger, the sympathetic system kicks in, increasing heart rate and blood flow to muscles, preparing the body to confront or escape the threat. This response is crucial for survival but can be detrimental if activated too frequently in our modern lives, leading to chronic stress and anxiety.

The third circuit, the ventral vagal complex, is unique to mammals and supports the social engagement system. This circuit regulates facial expressions, vocalizations, and social behaviors, facilitating connection and communication with others. When the ventral vagal complex is active, individuals feel safe and are more likely to engage in social interactions, fostering bonds and community. This system plays a vital role in emotional regulation.

Understanding these circuits offers practical insights into managing mental and physical health. For example, activating the ventral vagal complex through social interactions or calming practices can help mitigate stress and anxiety. Engaging in activities that promote safety and connection, such as spending time with loved ones or practicing mindfulness, can stimulate the ventral vagal complex, enhancing emotional resilience. This theory also provides a framework for addressing trauma and PTSD. By recognizing how the dorsal vagal complex's immobilization response manifests in trauma survivors, therapists can tailor interventions to gradually shift individuals towards the more adaptive ventral vagal state.

Scientific research supports the practical applications of Polyvagal Theory. For instance, studies in neurophysiology have shown that vagus nerve stimulation can improve heart rate variability, a marker of autonomic flexibility and resilience. Clinical applications in psychotherapy have demonstrated the benefits of incorporating Polyvagal Theory principles. Therapists use techniques that promote safety and social engagement to help clients move from hyperarousal or dissociation to states of calm and connection.

Incorporating Polyvagal Theory into daily life can transform how we manage stress and build emotional resilience. Simple practices such as deep breathing, gentle yoga, and spending time in nature can activate the ventral vagal complex. These activities promote relaxation and enhance social engagement, improving mental and physical health. The theory provides a solid basis for understanding why these practices work, offering a roadmap for achieving greater well-being.

CHAPTER 1

COMMON MISCONCEPTIONS ABOUT THE VAGUS NERVE

There are several misconceptions about the vagus nerve and its stimulation that need to be addressed. One of the most pervasive myths is that vagus nerve stimulation (VNS) is only helpful in treating epilepsy. While it is true that VNS has been FDA-approved for epilepsy since 1997, its benefits extend far beyond this condition. VNS has shown promise in treating depression, anxiety, and even inflammatory diseases. Research has demonstrated that stimulating the vagus nerve can reduce inflammation, enhance mood, and improve heart rate variability. These findings suggest that VNS can be an effective tool to manage and remedy a wide range of health issues, not just epilepsy.

Another common myth is that vagus nerve exercises are unsafe. This misconception mainly stems from a lack of understanding and fear of the unknown. In reality, vagus nerve exercises, such as deep breathing and gentle yoga, are safe and non-invasive. They are designed to be easily incorporated into daily routines without requiring special equipment or extensive training. Various cultures have used these practices for centuries to promote relaxation and well-being. Numerous studies have confirmed their safety and efficacy, making them accessible and beneficial for most people.

Understanding vagal tone is crucial for appreciating the vagus nerve's role in health. Vagal tone describes the activity of the vagus nerve and its effect on heart rate variability (HRV). High vagal tone is associated with a healthy, resilient autonomic nervous system. It is linked to better stress management and improved digestion. A common misconception is that vagal tone cannot be improved. However, research has shown that vagal tone can be enhanced through regular practice of specific exercises, such as deep breathing, meditation, and cold exposure. These practices stimulate the vagus nerve, promoting its activity and improving vagal tone over time.

Another misunderstanding is the belief that vagus nerve exercises lack scientific backing. This could not be further from the truth. Evidence supports the benefits of vagus nerve stimulation and exercises. For instance, a study found that stimulating the vagus nerve reduced inflammation and improved outcomes in patients with rheumatoid arthritis. Another study demonstrated that deep breathing exercises increased vagal tone and reduced anxiety. These findings underscore the broad health benefits of vagus nerve stimulation and validate the effectiveness of these practices.

Some people believe that the benefits of vagus nerve exercises are exaggerated. They may think these practices are too simple to significantly impact one's health. However, the simplicity of these exercises does not diminish their effectiveness. Deep breathing, mindfulness meditation, and gentle yoga may seem straightforward, but they profoundly affect the body's physiology. By regularly practicing these exercises, individuals can make big improvements in their mental and physical health. The key is consistency and commitment to integrating these practices into daily life.

In conclusion, debunking myths and clarifying misconceptions about the vagus nerve is essential for understanding its role in health. Vagus nerve stimulation is not limited to epilepsy; it offers broad health benefits supported by scientific evidence. Vagus nerve exercises are safe and effective, capable of improving vagal tone and enhancing overall well-being.

CHAPTER 2
SCIENTIFIC BACKING AND EVIDENCE

RESEARCH STUDIES ON VAGUS NERVE STIMULATION

The scientific community has done extensive research on the effects of vagus nerve stimulation (VNS) on health, yielding promising results. One of the most significant studies was conducted by Dr. Kevin Tracey, who explored the anti-inflammatory effects of VNS. His research demonstrated that stimulating the vagus nerve could significantly reduce inflammation. This reduction occurs through the cholinergic anti-inflammatory pathway, where the vagus nerve signals immune cells to release fewer pro-inflammatory cytokines. This finding opened new avenues for treating conditions like rheumatoid arthritis and inflammatory bowel disease, providing hope for many patients.

Another important area of research focuses on the impact of VNS on heart rate variability (HRV). HRV helps measure the variation in time between each heartbeat, reflecting the heart's ability to respond to stress. Higher HRV is linked with better cardiovascular health and greater resilience to stress. Studies have shown that VNS can increase HRV, promoting better autonomic nervous system balance. One particular study analyzed the effect of VNS on HRV during different states, such as sleep and wakefulness. The results indicated that VNS increased HRV complexity during sleep, suggesting enhanced parasympathetic activity and improved heart function.

To ensure the reliability of these findings, researchers employed rigorous methodologies. Randomized controlled trials (RCTs) are the gold standard in clinical research. They involve randomly assigning participants to either the treatment group or a control group, minimizing bias and ensuring that the results are attributable to the intervention. Longitudinal studies, which follow participants over an extended period, provide insights into the long-term effects of VNS. Cross-sectional analyses, on the other hand, compare different groups at a single point in time, offering a snapshot of the intervention's impact. Animal models are often used to explore the underlying mechanisms of VNS, while human clinical trials validate these findings in real-world settings.

The findings from these studies are compelling. Dr. Tracey's research revealed a significant reduction in inflammatory markers, such as cytokines, in patients practicing VNS. This reduction translates to decreased symptoms and a higher quality of life for people with chronic inflammatory conditions. Additionally, studies on HRV have shown that VNS improves HRV metrics and enhances mental health outcomes. Participants reported reduced anxiety and depression levels, highlighting the broader benefits of VNS beyond physical health.

Research also indicates enhanced gastrointestinal function through VNS. Studies have demonstrated improvements in conditions like irritable bowel syndrome (IBS) and gastroparesis. By stimulating the vagus nerve, VNS promotes better digestion and reduces gastrointestinal symptoms, relieving many patients suffering from these debilitating conditions. The application of VNS in these areas underscores its potential as a versatile therapeutic tool.

Visual representations are a great tool to help you understand the impact of VNS. Imagine a graph showing changes in HRV before and after VNS treatment. The upward trend in HRV reflects enhanced autonomic balance and improved heart health. Similarly, a table summarizing reductions in inflammatory cytokines provides a clear picture of the anti-inflammatory effects of VNS. These visual aids make the scientific data more accessible and relatable.

The scientific evidence supporting VNS is robust and multifaceted. From managing inflammation to improving heart rate variability and enhancing gastrointestinal function, VNS offers a range of health benefits validated by rigorous research. By understanding these studies, you can appreciate the foundation behind the practices you will learn in this book.

NEUROPLASTICITY AND THE VAGUS NERVE: EMERGING INSIGHTS

Imagine a young woman named Emily who struggled with cognitive decline after a traumatic brain injury. She found it difficult to focus, her memory was unreliable, and her overall cognitive function had diminished. Her life took a turn for the better when she started incorporating vagus nerve exercises into her daily routine. Over time, Emily began to notice significant improvements in her cognitive abilities. This transformation is rooted in neuroplasticity, the brain's amazing ability to reorganize and form new neural connections throughout life.

Neuroplasticity is the brain's capacity to adapt and change in response to experience, learning, or injury. This adaptive feature of the nervous system allows it to rewire itself, forming new connections and pathways that can compensate for lost functions or enhance existing ones. The concept of neuroplasticity underscores that the brain is not a static organ but a dynamic system capable of growth and transformation. This plasticity is vital for recovery from neurological injuries, adapting to new learning experiences, and maintaining cognitive health as we age.

Research shows that vagus nerve stimulation (VNS) can significantly influence neuroplasticity. One study focused on the role of VNS in promoting neurogenesis, the process through which new neurons are formed in the brain. The findings revealed that VNS could enhance neurogenesis, particularly in the hippocampus, a region critical for memory and learning. This suggests that regular vagus nerve stimulation can foster new neurons' growth, potentially improving cognitive functions affected by injury or age.

In addition to promoting neurogenesis, VNS has been shown to impact synaptic plasticity, which is the ability of synapses (the connections between neurons) to strengthen or weaken over time. Synaptic plasticity is fundamental for learning and memory functions. Research has demonstrated that VNS can enhance long-term potentiation (LTP), a process that strengthens the synapses involved in learning and memory. VNS can improve cognitive functions such as attention, problem-solving, and memory retention by boosting synaptic plasticity.

The implications of these findings are profound. Enhancing neuroplasticity through VNS holds significant potential for treating neurological disorders. For instance, individuals with conditions like Alzheimer's disease, stroke, or traumatic brain injuries could benefit from therapies that incorporate VNS to stimulate neurogenesis and synaptic plasticity. This approach could help restore cognitive functions and improve the quality of life for those affected by neurological impairments. Moreover, the cognitive enhancements associated with VNS could also benefit healthy individuals looking to maintain or boost their mental acuity as they age.

One compelling case study involved a middle-aged man named David, who experienced cognitive decline due to early-onset Alzheimer's disease. After integrating VNS into his treatment plan, David showed marked improvements in cognitive function. His memory and problem-solving skills improved, allowing him to regain some independence in his daily life. This real-life example highlights the potential of VNS to support cognitive health and recovery.

The link between vagus nerve stimulation (VNS) and neuroplasticity offers promising potential for boosting cognitive abilities and addressing neurological conditions. Stimulating the vagus nerve can encourage the growth of new neurons and reinforce synaptic connections, which may enhance mental clarity, memory, and learning skills. This emerging insight into neuroplasticity underscores the transformative potential of VNS in fostering brain health and cognitive resilience.

HEART RATE VARIABILITY: MEASURING VAGAL TONE

Heart rate variability (HRV) is a fascinating and vital measure of your heart's ability to adapt to various stressors. Essentially, HRV is the variation in time between each heartbeat, reflecting the dynamic interplay between your sympathetic and parasympathetic nervous systems. Higher HRV indicates a healthy, adaptable heart, while lower HRV can signal stress or potential health issues. The vagus nerve is essential for regulating heart rate variability (HRV), as it supports the balance between the two sections of the autonomic nervous system.

When your vagal tone is strong, your HRV tends to be higher, signaling better overall health and resilience. Several methodologies are employed to measure HRV, each offering unique insights into your autonomic function. One of the most common and accurate methods is the electrocardiogram (ECG), which records the electrical activity of your heart. ECGs provide a detailed picture of your HRV by analyzing the intervals between heartbeats. However, wearable HRV monitors have become increasingly popular for everyday use. Devices like heart rate belts and smartwatches can continuously track your heart rate and calculate HRV, making it convenient to monitor changes in real time. Another valuable tool is HRV biofeedback devices, which measure HRV and provide feedback to help you improve it through guided breathing exercises.

HRV is more than just a number; it's an accurate indicator of your overall health.. High HRV is associated with better stress resilience, meaning your body can effectively handle and recover from stress. This resilience is crucial for mental and emotional stability. Moreover, HRV is linked to cardiovascular health and longevity. Studies have shown that people with higher HRV usually have lower risks of heart disease and live longer healthier lives. Therefore, monitoring and improving HRV can be a proactive way to enhance your health and extend your lifespan.

Research has demonstrated the positive impact of vagus nerve exercises on HRV. By taking slow, deep breaths, you can stimulate the vagus nerve, which in turn enhances parasympathetic activity and boosts HRV. This practice can be particularly beneficial during stressful situations, helping you calm down and maintain physiological balance. Another compelling example comes from a woman named Rachel, who struggled with chronic stress and anxiety. By incorporating regular mindfulness and deep breathing exercises into her daily routine, Rachel markedly improved her HRV. This change translated to better emotional regulation and reduced anxiety, illustrating the real-life benefits of these simple practices.

Visualizing the impact of HRV can be incredibly insightful. Imagine a graph that tracks HRV before and after engaging in vagus nerve exercises. The upward trend in HRV post-exercise would clearly show the positive effects of these practices on your autonomic balance. Similarly, a table summarizing research findings on HRV improvements through various exercises can provide a concise overview of the benefits. These visual aids help you see the tangible results of incorporating vagus nerve exercises into your life.

The connection between HRV and vagal tone underscores the importance of monitoring and improving HRV for better health. By understanding how to measure HRV and the significance of this metric, you can take proactive steps to enhance your well-being. Simple practices like deep breathing, mindfulness, and regular use of HRV biofeedback devices can make a substantial difference.

EVIDENCE FROM CLINICAL TRIALS: WHAT SCIENCE SAYS

Clinical trials have been crucial in validating the effectiveness of vagus nerve stimulation (VNS) for various health conditions. One noteworthy trial focused on the use of VNS for treating depression, particularly treatment-resistant depression (TRD). This trial involved a randomized controlled design where people were divided into two groups: one received VNS while the other received a placebo treatment. The results were promising. Participants in the VNS group showed significant decreases in depression symptoms when compared to the placebo group. Long-term follow-up studies further confirmed these findings, revealing tangible improvements in mood and quality of life. These outcomes highlight the potential of VNS as an effective treatment option for people battling depression that doesn't respond to conventional therapies.

Another significant clinical trial examined the efficacy of VNS in managing epilepsy. This study also used a randomized controlled trial (RCT) design, which is regarded as the gold standard in clinical research. Participants were randomly assigned to either a VNS treatment group or a control group receiving standard epilepsy care. The trial's outcome measures included seizure frequency, severity, and overall quality of life. The results were remarkable. Patients receiving VNS experienced a substantial reduction in seizure frequency and severity, leading to improved daily functioning and quality of life. The long-term follow-up data supported these findings, showing the enduring benefits of VNS in epilepsy management.

The methodologies employed in these trials were rigorous and designed to ensure the reliability of the results. Randomized controlled trials with placebo groups minimize bias and establish a clear cause-and-effect relationship between the intervention and the observed outcomes. Long-term follow-up studies are crucial for assessing the durability of treatment effects over time. These studies often span several years, providing valuable insights into the long-term benefits and potential side effects of VNS. Outcome measures in these trials typically include symptom reduction, quality of life improvements, and overall health metrics, offering a comprehensive evaluation of the treatment's efficacy.

The practical implications of these clinical trials are far-reaching. The findings suggest that VNS can be integrated into mental health treatment plans for conditions like depression, particularly for patients who have not found relief through traditional methods. The robust evidence supporting VNS for epilepsy management also opens new avenues for improving the lives of those affected by this condition. Beyond these specific applications, VNS shows promise in managing chronic pain and inflammation, further broadening its therapeutic potential.

Visual aids can help illustrate the impact of VNS in these clinical trials. Imagine a graph showing the reduction in depressive symptoms over time for patients receiving VNS compared to those in the placebo group. The downward trend in depressive scores for the VNS group vividly depicts the treatment's effectiveness. Similarly, a table summarizing the quality of life improvements among epilepsy patients provides a clear picture of the benefits. These visual representations make the clinical data more accessible and relatable.

The evidence from these clinical trials underscores the transformative potential of VNS in treating various health conditions. By demonstrating significant improvements in symptoms and quality of life, these studies validate the effectiveness of VNS and highlight its practical applications in real-world settings. Whether for managing depression, epilepsy, or chronic pain, VNS offers a promising therapeutic option backed by rigorous research.

As we move forward, it's essential to consider the broader implications of these findings. The potential for VNS to improve mental and physical health is vast, and ongoing research continues to uncover new applications and benefits.

CHAPTER 3
MENTAL HEALTH HEALING EXERCISES

ALLEVIATING ANXIETY THROUGH VAGUS NERVE EXERCISES

The relationship between vagus nerve stimulation and anxiety relief is rooted in the parasympathetic nervous system's role in calming the body. When you activate the vagus nerve, it sends signals that help disengage the fight-or-flight response, reducing the stress hormones in your body. This shift promotes relaxation and restores balance. The vagus nerve's influence on heart rate variability (HRV) is crucial here. Higher HRV, associated with good vagal tone, indicates your body's ability to adapt to stress. By improving vagal tone through specific exercises, you can enhance HRV and better manage anxiety.

One effective vagus nerve exercise is deep **Diaphragmatic Breathing**:

1. Find a comfortable position, either lying down or sitting.
2. Put one hand on your chest and the other on your abdomen.

3. Take a slow, deep breath through your nose, and let your abdomen rise while keeping your chest still.
4. Exhale slowly through your mouth, and let the abdomen fall.
5. Repeat this for 5-10 minutes daily.

This technique stimulates the vagus nerve and encourages a state of relaxation.

Another powerful practice is **Progressive Muscle Relaxation**:

1. Begin by sitting or lying down in a quiet space.
2. Close your eyes and take a deep breath.
3. Tense the muscles as tightly as possible, starting with your feet.
4. After a few seconds, release.
5. Move up through the body, tensing and relaxing each muscle group.

This systematic relaxation helps reduce physical tension and anxiety, engaging the vagus nerve to promote calmness.

These exercises offer simple yet powerful tools to alleviate anxiety. By incorporating deep diaphragmatic breathing and progressive muscle relaxation into your daily routine, you can stimulate your vagus nerve and promote a state of relaxation. Whether you're dealing with social anxiety, workplace stress, or general anxiety, these exercises can help you find calm and balance in your life.

COMBATING DEPRESSION: TECHNIQUES AND PRACTICES

Depression is more than just feeling sad; it involves a complex mix of physiological and psychological factors. One significant factor is poor vagal tone, which can contribute to depressive symptoms. The vagus nerve plays a crucial role in regulating neurotransmitters like serotonin and norepinephrine, which impact mood. When the vagal tone is low, the balance of these neurotransmitters can be disrupted, leading to mood disturbances. Additionally, chronic inflammation has been linked to depression. The vagus nerve helps control the inflammatory response, and poor vagal tone can result in elevated inflammation levels, further exacerbating depressive symptoms.

To combat depression, several techniques can be highly effective. One such technique is heart rate variability (HRV) biofeedback. This method involves using a device to monitor your HRV and guide you through exercises that improve it. By practicing controlled breathing and focusing on the feedback, you can enhance your vagal tone and stabilize your mood. Another powerful approach is cold exposure therapy. Taking cold showers or immersing yourself in cold water can stimulate the vagus nerve, increasing neurotransmitter release and reducing inflammation. Gradually incorporating cold exposure into your routine can significantly improve your mental health.

Mindfulness and meditation are also key practices for improving vagus nerve function and easing depression symptoms. By concentrating on the present moment without judgment, mindfulness meditation encourages relaxation.

LOVING-KINDNESS MEDITATION: EMOTIONAL HEALING

Loving-kindness meditation, often called "metta" meditation, is a practice centered on cultivating feelings of compassion and kindness towards oneself and others. This type of meditation is about focusing on positive emotions, which can significantly impact your emotional health and enhance vagus nerve function. By engaging in loving-kindness meditation, you stimulate the parasympathetic nervous system, creating a sense of calm. This practice fosters emotional resilience and strengthens social connections, making it a powerful tool for overall mental health.

The **Loving-Kindness Meditation**:

1. Find a comfortable position.
2. Sit with your back straight, either on a chair or floor pillow and gently close your eyes.
3. Start by taking a few deep breaths to center yourself.
4. Then, silently repeat phrases of goodwill and compassion towards yourself, such as "May I be happy, may I be healthy, may I be safe."
5. Focus on these words and the feelings they evoke.
6. After a few minutes, expand your focus to include a loved one.
7. Picture them in your mind and repeat the same phrases, wishing them happiness, health, safety, and ease.
8. Gradually, extend this circle of compassion to include friends, family, acquaintances, and eventually all beings.

As you do this, try to genuinely feel the compassion and kindness you are sending out.

The benefits of loving-kindness meditation are profound. Practicing this meditation regularly can enhance feelings of compassion and empathy, allowing you to connect deeply with others. It helps reduce negative emotions such as anger, resentment, and frustration, promoting a positive outlook on life. Loving-kindness meditation improves social connections and builds emotional resilience by fostering a sense of emotional well-being. These benefits are closely linked to enhanced vagal tone, which supports better heart rate variability and overall health.

Studies have shown that loving-kindness meditation can nurture positive emotions and decrease depression symptoms, improving overall emotional health. This practice helps individuals manage stress more effectively and maintain positive social connections, contributing to overall mental health.

Practicing loving-kindness meditation regularly can cultivate a sense of compassion and kindness that enhances your emotional health and strengthens your vagus nerve function. This practice is a powerful healing tool, offering profound benefits for both mind and body.

MANAGING STRESS: DAILY VAGUS NERVE ROUTINES

Chronic stress can wreak havoc on your vagus nerve, impairing its function and throwing your autonomic nervous system out of balance. When you're constantly stressed, your body remains in a heightened state of alert, dominated by the sympathetic "fight or flight" response. Over time, this can weaken your vagal tone, making it harder for your body to return to a state of calm. Poor vagal tone can lead to a host of long-term health problems, including heart disease, digestive issues, and impaired immune function. Chronic stress is more than only a mental burden; it has real, detrimental effects on your physical health.

Implementing daily routines to manage stress can significantly improve your vagal tone. Start your day with morning breathing exercises. Find a quiet spot, sit comfortably, and take slow, deep breaths. Focus on the rise and fall of your abdomen as you breathe in through your nose and out through your mouth. This simple practice can set a calm tone for your day. Midday mindfulness breaks are another powerful tool. Take five to ten minutes to step away from your tasks. Find a quiet space, close your eyes, and focus on your breath. You can Listen to calming nature sounds to help you disconnect.

These short breaks can help reset your nervous system, reducing accumulated stress. In the evening, incorporate relaxation techniques to wind down. Try a gentle yoga session or guided imagery meditation. These practices can help you transition from the busyness of the day to a peaceful night.

Integrating these routines into your daily life offers numerous benefits. Improved heart rate variability is one of the most significant advantages, indicating better autonomic balance and resilience to stress. Enhanced emotional resilience is another key benefit, as regular vagus nerve exercises make managing emotional ups and downs easier. You'll likely find yourself feeling more grounded, focused, and capable of handling anything life throws your way.

Consistency is crucial for reaping these benefits. Set reminders on your phone to prompt you to take your mindfulness breaks. Use apps designed to guide you through breathing exercises and meditations. Create a supportive environment at home or work by designating a quiet space. Incorporate these routines into your daily life as essential habits, much like brushing your teeth or having your meals. With consistent effort, you'll experience a noticeable reduction in stress.

THE POWER OF HUMMING AND CHANTING IN STRESS MANAGEMENT

Humming and chanting are powerful tools that can significantly impact your stress levels by stimulating the vagus nerve. When you hum or chant, the vibrations in your throat and upper chest resonate through your body. These vibrations have a calming effect on your nervous system. The resonance produced by these activities helps to stimulate the vagus nerve, promoting relaxation and reducing stress. This stimulation enhances the parasympathetic nervous system's activity, which calms the body and restores balance.

The benefits of humming and chanting extend beyond immediate relaxation. These practices can increase your vagal tone, which is a measure of the health and activity of your vagus nerve. Higher vagal tone is associated with better emotional regulation, resilience to stress, and overall well-being. You may notice an enhanced sense of calmness when you practice humming or chanting. This is because these activities help to lower stress hormones like cortisol and increase the production of endorphins, the body's natural feel-good chemicals.

To start, try humming while exhaling. Find a comfortable position and take a deep breath through your nose. As you exhale slowly, hum in a steady tone. Feel the vibrations in your chest and throat. Repeat this for several minutes, focusing on the soothing sensation. Another effective practice is chanting simple mantras like "Om" or "Aum." Sit comfortably, inhale deeply, and chant the mantra as you exhale. The vibrations from chanting can help to deepen your relaxation. You can also use specific vowel sounds, such as "Ah" or "Ee," which produce different resonances in your body.

These exercises can be applied in various situations. During moments of acute stress, such as before a presentation or during a challenging day, take a few minutes to hum or chant. As a daily ritual, incorporate these practices into your morning or evening routine to set a calming tone for your day or promote restful sleep. Combining humming or chanting with other relaxation techniques, like deep breathing or meditation, can enhance their effectiveness.

LAUGHTER YOGA: USING JOY TO STIMULATE THE VAGUS NERVE

Laughter yoga combines the powerful benefits of laughter with the deep breathing techniques of yoga. Originated by Dr. Madan Kataria in 1995, this practice is grounded in the principles of unconditional laughter—laughing without relying on humor or jokes. Dr. Kataria discovered that the body cannot differentiate between real and simulated laughter, thus producing the same physiological and psychological benefits regardless of intent.

Laughter yoga has several remarkable benefits. When you laugh, your body releases endorphins and serotonin, the natural feel-good chemicals. This release helps to elevate your mood and create a sense of happiness. Laughter also reduces cortisol levels, the stress hormone, which helps you feel more relaxed and less anxious. By stimulating the vagus nerve, laughter yoga can improve heart rate variability and enhance your body's ability to recover from stress. The overall effect is an improvement in emotional well-being, making you feel more balanced and joyful.

To practice laughter yoga, start with some warm-up exercises. Begin by clapping your hands and chanting "Ho Ho, Ha Ha" rhythmically. This simple activity helps to loosen up and prepare for more intense laughter exercises. Next, engage in simulated laughter exercises like lion laughter, where you stick your tongue out and roar with laughter, or silent laughter, where you laugh without making a sound. These exercises can be done alone or in a group. Follow these with deep breathing and relaxation techniques to calm the body and mind. Conclude your session with a cool-down period and reflection to absorb the positive energy generated during the practice.

Integrating laughter yoga into your daily life can be both fun and beneficial. Consider joining a laughter yoga club or participating in online sessions to practice with others. If you're short on time, incorporate short laughter exercises during breaks at work. Use laughter yoga as a morning ritual to start your day with positivity or as an evening practice to unwind before bed. The flexibility of laughter yoga makes it easy to fit into any schedule, enhancing your overall well-being through the simple act of laughing.

SINGING AND ITS EFFECTS ON VAGAL TONE AND MOOD

Imagine a woman named Emily who found solace in singing. She discovered that the simple act of singing her favorite songs could profoundly impact her mood. This isn't surprising when you understand the physiological effects of singing on the vagus nerve. When you sing, vibrations in your vocal cords and the resonance in your chest create a calming effect. These vibrations stimulate the vagus nerve, activating the parasympathetic nervous system, which can help your body calm down. Additionally, singing triggers the release of oxytocin and endorphins, which are natural mood enhancers. This combination can help you feel more relaxed and uplifted.

Singing offers significant mental health benefits. Regular singing sessions can alleviate symptoms of depression by improving social connectedness and support. When you sing, you often do so with others, whether in a choir or a casual group, fostering a sense of community. This social activity can reduce feelings of isolation and loneliness. Singing also allows for emotional expression and release, providing an outlet for pent-up emotions that might otherwise contribute to depression. Engaging in this joyful activity can enhance your emotional health.

To incorporate singing into your routine, start with practical exercises. Sing your favorite songs or hymns daily, allowing yourself to get lost in the music. Practicing vocal scales and warm-ups can also be beneficial, as these exercises help improve your vocal technique and increase the calming vibrations in your body. Participating in choir groups or singing classes can provide additional social benefits and support. If joining a group isn't feasible, consider using apps or online platforms for guided singing sessions, which can help you stay motivated and be consistent.

Real-life examples highlight the transformative power of singing. Choir members often report increased happiness and reduced stress levels. Music therapy sessions have also shown promising results. Case studies reveal that patients with various mental health conditions experienced significant improvements in mood and emotional stability through structured singing exercises.

Emotional regulation is the foundation of mental health, influencing how you interact with the world and handle life's challenges. By stimulating your vagus nerve, you can gain better control over your emotions and improve your relationships.

CHAPTER 3

Mental Health
Vagus Nerve Exercises
Video Guide

CHAPTER 4
PHYSICAL HEALTH HEALING EXERCISES

CHRONIC PAIN RELIEF: TARGETED VAGUS NERVE TECHNIQUES

Chronic pain often feels like an uninvited guest that overstays its welcome, affecting your quality of life. The vagus nerve plays a big part in pain perception and modulation. When your vagal tone is impaired, your body's ability to manage pain diminishes. This nerve influences how pain signals are processed in your brain, meaning a low vagal tone can make you more sensitive to pain. Additionally, the vagus nerve helps regulate inflammatory markers in your body. Poor vagal tone can increase inflammation, exacerbating chronic pain conditions.

Specific vagus nerve exercises can be incredibly effective in alleviating chronic pain. Gentle yoga poses, for instance, can offer targeted pain relief.

Poses like **Child's Pose (Balasana)** and **Cat-Cow Pose (Marjaryasana-Bitilasana)** help stretch and relax muscles without putting too much strain on your body:

HEALING WITH VAGUS NERVE EXERCISES

1. Begin by finding a quiet space and laying out a yoga mat.
2. Start with Child's Pose by kneeling on the mat, sitting back on your heels, and stretching your arms forward while lowering your forehead to the ground.
3. Hold this position for a few minutes, focusing on your breath.
4. Transition into Cat-Cow Pose by moving onto all fours.
5. Inhale & arch your back (Cow Pose).
6. Exhale & round your back (Cat Pose).
7. Repeat for several breaths.

Deep breathing techniques also provide immediate pain reduction. **Diaphragmatic Breathing,** for example, can help calm your nervous system:

1. Sit comfortably.
2. Place a hand on your chest and the other on your abdomen.
3. Inhale through your nose & let your abdomen rise more than your chest.
4. Exhale slowly through your mouth.
5. Repeat this for a few minutes to stimulate your vagus nerve & reduce pain.

Mindfulness Practices further enhance vagal tone and alleviate pain. This type of meditation involves focusing on the present without judgment, which can help you manage pain more effectively:

1. Find a quiet space, sit comfortably, and close your eyes.
2. Focus on your breath, noticing the sensation of air entering & leaving your body.
3. If you get distracted, gently bring your focus back to your breath.

CHAPTER 4

Body Scan Meditation is another powerful tool:

1. Lie down comfortably and close your eyes.
2. Starting from your toes, slowly bring awareness to each part of your body.
3. Be aware of any tension or discomfort.
4. As you focus on each area, imagine releasing the tension with each exhale.

Real-life case studies illustrate the effectiveness of these practices. Consider Maria, who suffered from fibromyalgia. By incorporating gentle yoga and mindfulness meditation into her routine, Maria experienced a significant reduction in her pain levels. She found that these practices alleviated her physical discomfort and improved her mental state.

Understanding the connection between vagus nerve health and chronic pain can empower you to take control of your recovery. You can improve your vagal tone and alleviate chronic pain through targeted exercises like gentle yoga, deep breathing, and mindfulness practices.

ACUPRESSURE POINTS FOR VAGAL STIMULATION AND PAIN RELIEF

Acupressure, rooted in Traditional Chinese Medicine (TCM), is an ancient practice that involves applying pressure to specific points on the body to activate healing and relieve pain. This technique works on the principle that stimulating certain points can influence the flow of energy, or "qi," along the body's meridians. By doing so, acupressure can enhance the function of the vagus nerve, which is crucial for regulating pain and promoting relaxation. Pressure points are believed to communicate with the body's nervous system, sending signals that can modulate pain perception and reduce inflammation.

LI4:

One of the most effective acupressure points for vagal stimulation and pain relief is LI4, also known as Hegu. This point can be found between the thumb and index finger. This point helps alleviate headaches, stress, and pain. To find LI4, simply press the fleshy area between your thumb and index finger.

PC6:

Another vital point is PC6, or Neiguan, situated on the inner forearm, three finger widths from the wrist. This point is excellent for nausea, anxiety, and chest pain.

ST36:

ST36, or Zusanli, is located four finger widths below the knee and one finger width to the outside. It is beneficial for digestive issues and general pain relief.

GB20:

Lastly, GB20, or Fengchi, can be found at the base of the skull in the hollows on both sides of your neck. This point is effective for headaches, neck pain, and stress.

To apply **Acupressure**:

1. Start by locating the desired point accurately.
2. Use your fingers to gently apply pressure firmly.
3. Maintain the pressure for about 30 seconds to a minute, then release.
4. Repeat this process several times, ensuring you breathe deeply throughout the session.

For optimal results, acupressure sessions should be performed a few times a day. To enhance the effectiveness of acupressure, combine it with deep breathing exercises. This combination promotes greater relaxation and enhances vagal stimulation. Applying gentle heat to the area before starting can also make the session more effective. Acupressure tools like a massage ball can help apply more precise pressure.

Through regular practice, you can harness the benefits of acupressure to stimulate your vagus nerve and alleviate pain. This ancient technique offers a simple yet powerful way to manage discomfort.

REDUCING INFLAMMATION: HOLISTIC METHODS

The vagus nerve helps regulate inflammation within the body. When the vagus nerve is stimulated, it activates an anti-inflammatory pathway that helps control the body's inflammatory response. This pathway influences the production of cytokines, proteins that signal inflammation. The vagus nerve can reduce inflammation and promote healing by modulating cytokine production. This mechanism is crucial for managing conditions like arthritis, autoimmune diseases, and chronic inflammation, which can lead to various health issues.

Cold exposure therapy is one effective method to stimulate the vagus nerve and reduce inflammation. This involves exposing your body to cold temperatures through cold showers or ice baths. The cold stimulates the vagus nerve, activating the anti-inflammatory pathway. Start with a brief cold shower, gradually increasing the duration as you become more comfortable. Resonant frequency breathing is another practical technique. By breathing at a specific rate, usually around five breaths per minute, you can stimulate the vagus nerve and reduce inflammation.

Resonant Frequency Breathing:

1. Sit comfortably.
2. Inhale deeply for a count of five.
3. Exhale for a count of five.
4. Continue this pattern for several minutes.

Diet and lifestyle significantly impact vagus nerve function and inflammation levels. An anti-inflammatory diet supplemented with fruits, vegetables, lean proteins, and healthy fats can support vagal tone. Foods like salmon, berries, and leafy greens are excellent choices. Regular physical activity also enhances vagus nerve function. Aim for at least 30 minutes of exercise three to 4 days of the week. Activities like walking, swimming, and yoga are beneficial.

Scientific research supports these methods. Studies on vagus nerve stimulation have shown significant reductions in inflammatory markers. For instance, clinical trials have demonstrated that dietary interventions can improve vagal tone and reduce inflammation. Practicing these exercises during the day can help you manage inflammation and improve overall health.

ANTI-INFLAMMATORY BREATHING TECHNIQUES

Anti-inflammatory breathing techniques offer a natural and effective way to reduce inflammation by stimulating the vagus nerve. These techniques activate the parasympathetic nervous system, helping to calm your body and mind. These breathing practices promote overall relaxation and stress reduction, further supporting your body in managing inflammation.

Nostril Breathing (Nadi Shodhana) is an effective technique:

1. Sit comfortably & close the right nostril with your thumb.
2. Inhale through the left nostril & close your left nostril.
3. Release your right nostril & exhale through it.

4. Inhale through the right nostril, close it, & exhale through the left.
5. Repeat this cycle for several minutes & stay focused on your breath.

Four-Square Breathing is another powerful method:

1. Sit comfortably & inhale deeply through your nose for four seconds.
2. Hold your breath for four seconds.
3. Exhale slowly through your mouth for a count of four, then pause and hold for a final count of four.
4. Repeat this process for a few minutes to stimulate the vagus nerve and reduce inflammation.

Coherent Breathing involves maintaining a steady breathing rate of about five breaths per minute:

1. Sit comfortably & inhale deeply for a count of five seconds, then exhale for five seconds.
2. Continue this pattern for several minutes while you focus on the rhythm of your breath.

This technique helps regulate your heart rate and enhances vagus nerve function.

Combining these exercises with mindfulness meditation can amplify their effects. Calming background music or nature sounds can also enhance your practice, creating a serene atmosphere supporting relaxation and healing.

GENTLE STRETCHING EXERCISES FOR ARTHRITIS RELIEF

Arthritis can be debilitating, causing joint stiffness and chronic pain that disrupts daily life. Gentle stretching exercises can significantly alleviate these symptoms by stimulating the vagus nerve, which helps alleviate pain and inflammation. Stretching enhances flexibility and increases the range of motion, making it easier to move without causing discomfort. As you stretch, your body releases tension, promoting relaxation and reducing stress. These exercises also support joint health by improving circulation and nutrient delivery to areas in need.

Begin with the **Cat-Cow Stretch (Marjaryasana-Bitilasana)**, which helps mobilize the spine and relieve tension:

1. Start on all fours.
2. Align your wrists under your shoulders & knees under your hips.
3. Inhale while arching your back (Cow Pose), lifting your head & tailbone.
4. Exhale while you round your spine (Cat Pose), tucking your chin and tailbone. Repeat this sequence for several breaths.

Next, the **Seated Forward Bend (Paschimottanasana)** stretches the hamstrings and lower back:

1. Sit with your legs extended.
2. Inhale & lengthen your spine.
3. Exhale as you reach forward, keeping your back straight.
4. Hold for a few breaths.

For the **Standing Hamstring Stretch**:

CHAPTER 4

1. Stand with your feet hip-width apart. Step one foot back, keeping both legs straight.
2. Bend at your hips and extend your reach toward your front foot, experiencing the stretch in your hamstring.
3. Hold for a few breaths before switching sides.

The **Shoulder Stretch** can be done by:

1. Place one arm horizontally across your chest.
2. Hold it with the opposite hand.

This stretch relieves shoulder tension and improves flexibility.

Lastly, **Wrist and Finger Stretches** are essential for those with arthritis in the hands:

1. Extend one arm in front.
2. Put your palm up & gently pull back on the fingers with the opposite hand.
3. Switch sides after a few breaths.

A guided stretching routine can further enhance the benefits. Begin with warm-up exercises like gentle neck rolls and shoulder shrugs. Move into the main stretches, focusing on each pose for several breaths. Incorporate deep breathing to stimulate the vagus nerve and promote relaxation. Finish with a cool-down period, doing light stretches and deep breathing. Practicing safely is crucial to avoid injury. Always listen to your body's signals and avoid pushing into pain. Use props like yoga blocks and straps for support, and practice in a comfortable, quiet environment.

BREATHING TECHNIQUES TO ENHANCE DIGESTIVE FUNCTION

Proper breathing techniques can significantly impact your digestive health by stimulating the vagus nerve. When you breathe deeply and rhythmically, you are activating the parasympathetic nervous system, which promotes relaxation and reduces stress. This activation enhances the production of digestive enzymes, essential for breaking down food and taking in nutrients. Additionally, it improves gut motility and peristalsis, which are the wave-like contractions that move food through your digestive tract. Proper breathing reduces gastrointestinal stress and discomfort, making digestion smoother and more efficient.

One effective breathing technique is **Pursed-Lip Breathing**:

1. Sit comfortably.
2. Inhale through your nose & count to four.
3. Purse your lips as if you are about to whistle, then exhale slowly and gently through your lips for a count of six.
4. Repeat this process for several minutes.

Resonant Breathing and **Diaphragmatic Breathing** are also great exercises to enhance digestion. To practice these techniques effectively:

1. Find a comfortable, seated position in a quiet environment.
2. Begin with a few deep, slow breaths to center yourself.
3. Practice each technique for five to ten minutes and gradually increase the duration as you become more comfortable.

Practicing these techniques before meals can stimulate digestion. Combine them with mindful eating practices to enhance the benefits, such as chewing slowly and savoring each bite. Using apps or guided audio can provide additional support and help you stay consistent with your practice.

YOGA POSES TO ALLEVIATE IBS SYMPTOMS

Yoga offers a holistic approach to managing irritable bowel syndrome (IBS) by stimulating the vagus nerve, which helps alleviate symptoms such as abdominal discomfort and bloating. Engaging in specific yoga poses enhances gut motility and peristalsis, the muscle contractions that move food through your digestive tract. Additionally, yoga promotes overall relaxation and stress reduction, which is essential for managing IBS. By improving the communication between your gut and brain, these practices can significantly alleviate IBS symptoms, creating a more harmonious internal environment.

One effective pose is **Cat-Cow Pose (Marjaryasana-Bitilasana)**. This pose helps massage your abdominal organs, improving gut motility:

1. Begin on all fours.
2. Line your wrists under your shoulders & knees under your hips.
3. Inhale & arch your back while you lift your head and tailbone (Cow Pose).
4. Start to exhale as you round your spine, tucking your chin and tailbone (Cat Pose).

Another beneficial pose is the **Seated Forward Bend (Paschimottanasana)**. This stretch aids in digestion and helps reduce bloating:

1. Sit with your legs extended.

2. Inhale to lengthen your spine.
3. Exhale as you reach forward, keeping your back straight.

Supine Twist (Supta Matsyendrasana) is excellent for stimulating the digestive organs:

1. Lay on your back.
2. Bring your knees to your chest.
3. Let them fall to one side while extending your arms out.
4. Hold for a few breaths before switching sides.

Child's Pose (Balasana) is another calming pose. This pose helps relax the body and mind, reducing stress-related IBS symptoms:

1. Kneel on the mat.
2. Sit back on your heels.
3. Stretch your arms forward & lower your forehead to the ground simultaneously.

Bridge Pose (Setu Bandhasana) stimulates the abdominal organs and improves digestion:

1. Lay on your back.
2. Bend your knees & keep your feet flat on the ground.
3. Lift your hips towards the sky & engage your core.

A guided yoga routine can further enhance these benefits. Start with light warm-up exercises to prepare your body. Move into the primary yoga poses, focusing on deep, rhythmic breathing. Conclude with a cool-down period, incorporating light stretches and relaxation techniques. Always listen to your body's signals and avoid pushing into pain. Use props like yoga blocks and straps for support, and practice in a comfortable, quiet environment to maximize the effectiveness of your session.

CHAPTER 4

Physical Health
Vagus Nerve Exercises Video Guide

CHAPTER 5
PTSD AND TRAUMA RECOVERY EXERCISES

GROUNDING TECHNIQUES FOR PTSD RELIEF

Grounding is a coping strategy that helps you stay connected to the present moment. It's particularly useful for managing PTSD symptoms, such as fear, anxiety, flashbacks, and dissociation. The mechanism behind grounding is simple yet powerful. By focusing on the here and now, you can interrupt distressing thoughts and bring your attention back to the present. This shift in focus not only reduces the intensity of PTSD symptoms but also helps stimulate the vagus nerve, producing a sense of calm and reducing overall anxiety.

One effective grounding technique is the **5-4-3-2-1 Method**, which uses your five senses to anchor you in the present:

1. Start by taking a deep breath.
2. Notice five things you can see around you.
3. Notice four things you can touch, such as the fabric of your clothes or the texture of a nearby object.

4. Follow this by noticing three things you can hear, like the refrigerator's hum or the distant sound of traffic.
5. Notice two things you can smell, whether it's the scent of your soap or the aroma of a nearby plant.
6. Finally, identify one thing you can taste, such as the lingering flavor of a recent meal.

This sensory exercise helps ground you, making you more aware of your surroundings and less focused on distressing thoughts.

Physical grounding involves using touch to connect with the present. This can be as simple as holding an object and focusing on its texture and temperature. For instance, you might hold a smooth stone or a piece of fabric, paying close attention to how it feels in your hand. Another method is to press your feet firmly into the ground and notice the sensation. These physical connections help anchor you in the present, reducing feelings of dissociation and anxiety.

Movement can also be a powerful grounding tool. Simple activities like walking, stretching, or even dancing can help you feel more connected to your body and the present moment. As you move, focus on the sensations in your body—the way your feet feel against the floor, the stretch in your muscles, or the rhythm of your movements. Focusing on physical sensations can help break the cycle of distressing thoughts and bring you back to the here and now.

Visualization Grounding involves imagining a safe and peaceful place:

1. Close your eyes and take a few deep breaths.
2. Picture a location where you feel completely at ease, whether it's a sunny beach, a quiet forest, or a cozy room.

3. Imagine the sights, sounds, smells, and textures of this place in vivid detail.

Spending a few minutes in this mental sanctuary can help reduce anxiety and provide a sense of safety and calm.

To practice grounding effectively, start by finding a quiet, comfortable space where you won't be disturbed. Begin with a few minutes of deep breathing to relax your body and mind. Choose one of the grounding techniques described above and move through it slowly, taking your time to fully engage with each step. After completing the exercise, take a moment to reflect on how you feel. Notice any changes in your level of anxiety or sense of presence. Conclude your session with a few more deep breaths to reinforce the sense of calm.

Practicing grounding regularly can enhance its effectiveness. Try to add these techniques into your daily routine, using them whenever you feel overwhelmed or disconnected. Grounding can be especially helpful during moments of acute stress, providing an immediate way to regain control and calm. Combining grounding with calming practices, such as deep breathing or mindfulness meditation, can enhance its benefits. Remember, the goal is to stay connected to the present moment, reducing the impact of distressing thoughts and promoting peace and stability.

DEEP BREATHING TO CALM THE NERVOUS SYSTEM

Deep breathing exercises are invaluable tools for calming the nervous system, particularly for individuals dealing with PTSD. These exercises stimulate the vagus nerve, which activates the parasympathetic nervous system. This part of the nervous system is tasked with counteracting the body's fight-or-flight response. When the parasympathetic system is engaged, it helps reduce hyperarousal and anxiety, creating a sense of calm and security. By practicing deep breathing regularly, you can teach your body to manage stress more effectively, decreasing the intensity of PTSD symptoms.

One effective deep breathing technique is **Box Breathing**. This method involves inhaling, holding your breath, exhaling, and pausing in a rhythmic pattern:

1. To start, find a comfortable position, either seated or lying down.
2. Close your eyes and inhale deeply through your nose for four seconds.
3. Hold your breath for another four seconds.
4. Exhale through your mouth for four seconds.
5. Pause and hold your breath again for four seconds.
6. Repeat this cycle several times.

This structured breathing pattern helps regulate your heart rate and promotes a calming effect on the nervous system.

Coherent Breathing is another powerful technique that involves breathing at a rate of five breaths per minute. This method aims to synchronize your breath with your heart rate, enhancing heart rate variability and promoting a state of relaxation. To practice coherent breathing:

1. Sit or lie down comfortably.
2. Inhale deeply through your nose for six seconds.
3. Exhale through your mouth for six seconds.
4. Continue this pattern for several minutes, focusing on your breath's smooth, steady rhythm.

Coherent breathing can be particularly effective in reducing anxiety.

The **4-7-8 Breathing** technique is also widely recognized for its calming effects:

1. Begin by finding a quiet, comfortable space.
2. Close your eyes and inhale deeply through your nose for four seconds.
3. Hold your breath for seven seconds.
4. Exhale through your mouth for eight seconds.
5. Repeat this cycle four times.
6. Gradually increase the number of repetitions as you become more comfortable with the practice.

The 4-7-8 breathing technique helps slow down your heart rate and calm the mind, making it an excellent tool for managing PTSD symptoms.

Creating a quiet, comfortable environment is essential to practicing deep breathing effectively. Find a peaceful space where you won't be disturbed, and consider using calming background music or nature sounds to enhance relaxation. Combining deep breathing with visualization or grounding techniques can further amplify its benefits. For example, while practicing box breathing, you might visualize a square, tracing its edges with each breath. Regular practice is vital to reap the full benefits of these techniques. Aim to incorporate deep breathing exercises into your daily routine, using them as a tool to manage stress.

SOMATIC EXPERIENCING AND VAGAL TONE

Somatic Experiencing (SE) is a therapeutic approach developed by Dr. Peter Levine that focuses on the body's sensations to help release trauma. It works by guiding individuals to gradually reconnect with their physical sensations. This process helps them release the tension and energy stored in their bodies due to traumatic experiences. SE is deeply connected to the functioning of the vagus nerve, which plays a big role in regulating bodily responses to stress and trauma. Stimulating the vagus nerve can engage the parasympathetic nervous system, facilitating relaxation and aiding in counteracting the impacts of trauma.

The principles of Somatic Experiencing revolve around the idea that trauma is stored in the body and can be released through awareness and gentle interventions. In SE, the focus is on bodily sensations rather than thoughts or emotions. By paying attention to the body's physical experiences, individuals can begin to release the trauma stored within. The vagus nerve is crucial in this process, as it helps regulate the body's stress response. When activated, it can help individuals move from a state of hyperarousal or shutdown to a state of calm and safety.

One of the primary benefits of SE for individuals with PTSD is the reduction in trauma-related stress and anxiety. By focusing on bodily sensations and using gentle techniques to release stored energy, SE can help alleviate the intense stress and anxiety that often accompany PTSD. This stress reduction can lead to improved emotional regulation and stability. When the vagus nerve is stimulated through SE, it can enhance the body's ability to manage emotional responses, leading to a greater sense of control and stability.

Practical SE exercises can be very effective in managing PTSD symptoms. One such technique is **Body Scanning** and awareness:

1. Rest in a lying or seated position and focus your attention on various areas of your body.
2. Become aware of any feelings or tension.
3. Start from your toes and work your way up to your head.
4. Take your time to observe each area.

CHAPTER 5

This practice helps you become more aware of your body and can reveal areas where trauma is stored.

Pendulation is another SE technique that involves alternating your focus between areas of comfort and discomfort in your body. This helps you manage the intensity of your sensations and prevents overwhelm:

1. Begin by noticing a part of your body that feels comfortable or neutral.
2. Spend a few moments focusing on this area before shifting your attention to a part that feels tense or uncomfortable.
3. Alternate between these areas, allowing yourself to return to the comfortable sensation whenever the discomfort becomes too intense.

Titration is the gradual exposure to traumatic memories in small, manageable doses. This technique helps prevent re-traumatization and allows the body to process trauma at its own pace:

1. Start by thinking of a mildly distressing memory and
2. Notice the sensations in your body.
3. Pay attention to your body's signals and take breaks as needed.

Over time, you can gradually increase the intensity of the memories you work with, allowing your body to release the trauma slowly.

Self-soothing techniques are also essential in SE. These might include gentle self-massage, holding a comforting object, or using a weighted blanket. These techniques help activate the vagus nerve and promote a sense of safety and calm. To practice SE safely, it's crucial to work with a trained SE practitioner if possible. They can guide you through the exercises and ensure you aren't overwhelmed. Always practice in a safe, supportive environment and listen to your body's signals. If you start to feel overwhelmed, take a break and return to a state of comfort before continuing.

SAFE TOUCH AND ITS IMPACT ON VAGAL HEALTH

Safe touch is a powerful tool for individuals with PTSD. It helps stimulate the vagus nerve and promotes a sense of safety and calm. The mechanism behind safe touch involves activating the parasympathetic nervous system, which fights against the body's stress responses. This activation can reduce hyperarousal and anxiety, allowing the body to relax and heal. When you engage in safe touch, your body releases oxytocin, often called the "love hormone." This hormone fosters feelings of trust and connection, further enhancing the sense of safety.

One effective safe touch practice is **Self-Hugging**:

1. Find a comfortable space to sit or lie down without interruptions.
2. Wrap your arms around yourself in a gentle hug, feeling the pressure and warmth of your own embrace.
3. Hold this position for a few minutes, focusing on the sensation of being held and supported.

This simple act can provide immediate comfort and stimulate the vagus nerve, helping to reduce anxiety and promote relaxation.

Another practice is **Self-Massage**:

1. Begin by sitting comfortably and using your hands to gently massage your shoulders, neck, and arms.
2. Pay attention to the pressure and movement of your hands, allowing yourself to focus on the physical sensations.

This can help ground you in the present moment and create a sense of calm. You might also try massaging your temples or the base of your skull, areas where tension often accumulates. Regular self-massage can enhance your body's ability to relax and reduce PTSD symptoms.

Gentle touch with a trusted person can also be incredibly healing. This might involve holding hands, receiving a hug, or simply sitting close to someone you trust. The presence of a loved one can amplify the calming effects of touch, creating a strong sense of safety and connection. It's important to communicate openly with your partner or friend about what feels comfortable and safe for you. Establishing clear boundaries ensures that the experience remains positive and supportive.

Using weighted blankets or body pillows can provide similar benefits. These tools apply gentle pressure to the body, mimicking the sensation of being held. This pressure can stimulate the vagus nerve and activate the parasympathetic nervous system. To use a weighted blanket, drape it over yourself while lying down, allowing the weight to distribute evenly. Focus on the sensation of the blanket's pressure, noticing how it helps your body relax. Body pillows can be used in a similar way, providing support and comfort during sleep or relaxation.

Engaging in therapeutic touch therapies, such as massage therapy, can be highly beneficial. Professional massage therapists are trained to use exercises that promote relaxation and stimulate the vagus nerve. Consistent sessions can help reduce muscle tension, improve circulation, and enhance overall well-being. If you decide to pursue massage therapy, choose a therapist who is experienced in working with individuals with PTSD. Communicate your needs and comfort levels to ensure a positive and healing experience.

To practice safe touch effectively, start by finding a quiet, comfortable environment where you feel secure. Begin with a few minutes of deep breathing to relax your body and mind. Choose a safe touch technique that feels right for you, whether it's self-hugging, self-massage, or using a weighted blanket. Apply a gentle, soothing touch, focusing on the sensations and allowing yourself to relax. Aim to practice safe touch regularly, incorporating it into your daily routine for best results. Combining safe touch with deep breathing or grounding techniques can further enhance its benefits. If you find it challenging to practice safe touch on your own, consider seeking help from a therapist who can guide you through the process.

CHAPTER 5

PTSD & Trauma
Vagus Nerve Exercises
Video Guide

CHAPTER 6
HOLISTIC WEIGHT LOSS EXERCISES

MINDFUL EATING AND ITS IMPACT ON VAGAL TONE

Mindful eating brings your full attention to the experience of eating. It encourages you to focus on the present moment, savoring each bite and recognizing your body's hunger and satiety cues. This practice can significantly enhance vagal tone, which is crucial for regulating digestion and metabolism. By engaging the parasympathetic nervous system, mindful eating helps shift the body from a state of stress to one of relaxation, promoting better digestive function.

Mindful eating allows you to truly experience the act of eating. This means being aware of your food's sight, smell, taste, and texture. By slowing down and chewing thoroughly, you give your body time to recognize when it is full, reducing the likelihood of overeating. Techniques such as pausing between bites and assessing your hunger levels can further enhance this awareness. Avoiding distractions like TV and smartphones during meals helps keep your focus on the food and your body's signals.

The upside of mindful eating for weight loss is manifold. By improving recognition of satiety signals, you are less likely to eat past the point of fullness. This can lead to a reducing your overall calorie intake without feeling deprived. Mindful eating also addresses emotional and binge eating by promoting a healthier relationship with food. Instead of using food as a coping mechanism for stress or boredom, you begin to enjoy meals for their nourishment and pleasure. Enhanced enjoyment and satisfaction from meals means you are more likely to feel content with smaller portions, which supports weight management.

To practice mindful eating, start by making a conscious effort to eat slowly. Chew each bite thoroughly and taste the flavors and textures. Engage all your senses: notice the vibrant colors of your vegetables, the aroma of fresh herbs, and the crunch of a crisp apple. Pause between bites to assess your hunger levels. Ask yourself if you are still hungry or eating out of habit. Create a peaceful eating environment by turning off the TV and putting away your phone. Focus only on your meal and the experience of eating.

There are real-life examples of individuals who have benefited from mindful eating. Take, for example, Angela, a marketing executive who struggled with late-night snacking. By practicing mindful eating, she learned to recognize her true hunger cues. She found that she was often eating out of boredom rather than hunger. Over time, Angela lost weight and felt more in control of her eating habits.

Starting mindful eating can change your relationship with food and support your weight loss goals. You can enhance vagal tone and promote better digestive health by focusing on present-moment awareness, savoring each bite, and recognizing your body's hunger and fullness cues. This simple practice can lead to positive benefits to your eating habits.

CHAPTER 6

BREATHING EXERCISES TO REDUCE EMOTIONAL EATING

Imagine you're in a quiet room, feeling the weight of the day's stress. Your mind races and the urge to reach for a snack becomes almost irresistible. Emotional eating often stems from a desire to cope with stress and anxiety. This is where the vagus nerve comes into play. By enhancing vagal tone, specific breathing exercises can help reduce emotional eating by activating the parasympathetic nervous system, which calms the body and mind. This shift from the "fight or flight" response to a state of relaxation can significantly reduce stress and anxiety levels, improving your ability to regulate emotions and cope with cravings more effectively.

One effective technique is the **4-7-8 Breathing** method. To begin:

1. Find a comfortable, seated position.
2. Close your eyes and place the tip of your tongue on the ridge of tissue just behind your upper front teeth.
3. Exhale entirely through your mouth.
4. Close your mouth and inhale slowly using your nose for four seconds.
5. Hold your breath for seven seconds.
6. Exhale through your mouth for eight seconds.

This simple sequence can help you regain control and reduce the urge to eat when your body is stressed.

Another method is **Resonant Breathing**. It involves breathing at a rate of five to six breaths per minute:

1. Inhale for six seconds.
2. Exhale for six seconds .

This breathing rhythm synchronizes your heart rate with your breathing, promoting a calm and balanced state.

Diaphragmatic Breathing, or **Deep Belly Breathing**, is another powerful tool:

1. Sit comfortably and place one hand on your chest and the other on your abdomen.
2. Inhale through your nose and let your abdomen rise more than your chest.
3. Exhale through your mouth, feeling your abdomen fall.

This exercise helps activate the vagus nerve and reduce anxiety.

For a guided breathing practice focused on reducing emotional eating, start by setting the scene. Find a quiet, comfortable place to sit. Close your eyes and focus on your breath. Begin with the 4-7-8 technique, repeating the sequence four times. Move on to coherent breathing, maintaining a steady rhythm of five breaths per minute for five minutes. Follow this with diaphragmatic breathing for another five minutes. Focus on the timing of your inhales, holds, and exhales. Practicing these techniques before meals can help reduce stress-induced cravings and promote mindful eating.

To make these breathing exercises more effective, consider combining them with mindfulness techniques. For instance, do a quick body scan after completing your breathing exercises. Close your eyes and bring your attention to different parts of your body. Notice any tension or discomfort.

Visualization can also enhance the practice. Picture a calm, serene place where you feel safe and relaxed. Using a breathing app or guided audio can provide additional support and structure to your practice, making it easier to stay consistent.

Incorporating these breathing exercises into your daily routine can significantly reduce emotional eating by enhancing vagal tone and promoting relaxation. Practicing before meals can create a buffer against stress-induced cravings and make more mindful, intentional choices about what and when to eat.

PHYSICAL ACTIVITY TO ENHANCE VAGAL HEALTH AND WEIGHT LOSS

Imagine stepping outside on a crisp morning, the air fresh and invigorating. You start with a brisk walk, feeling your body come alive with each step. Physical activity like this boosts your energy and enhances your vagal tone, which is crucial for your overall health. Regular exercise improves heart rate variability (HRV), a key indicator of autonomic nervous system balance. Higher HRV is linked to better stress management, reduced inflammation, and improved mental well-being. Participating in physical activity activates the parasympathetic nervous system, promoting relaxation and reducing the body's stress response.

Cardiovascular activities like walking, running, swimming, and cycling are especially beneficial for improving vagal health. These activities increase your heart rate in a controlled manner, improving cardiovascular health and boosting HRV. Walking is a simple yet powerful exercise. Aim for at least 30 minutes a day, whether it's a morning stroll or an evening walk. Jogging offers a more intense workout that can further enhance cardiovascular fitness. Start with short distances and gradually increase as your stamina improves.

Riding a bike, whether on a stationary model or outside, offers a great cardiovascular exercise that also builds leg strength. Strength training, including weight lifting and resistance bands, supports weight loss and enhances vagal tone. Building muscle increases your resting metabolic rate, letting your body burn more calories even at rest. Incorporate exercises such as squats, lunges, and deadlifts into your routine. Use resistance bands for added intensity and variety.

Try two to three weekly strength training sessions focusing on different muscle groups. Flexibility exercises like yoga and Pilates improve physical flexibility and enhance vagal tone. Yoga is particularly effective with its combination of physical postures, breath control, and meditation. Poses such as Downward Dog, Child's Pose, and Warrior II stimulate the vagus nerve and promote relaxation. Pilates, emphasizing core strength and controlled movements, also supports vagal health. Incorporate a 20-minute yoga or Pilates session into your daily routine to enjoy these benefits.

High-Intensity Interval Training (HIIT) offers a time-efficient and effective way to enhance vagal tone and support weight loss. HIIT exercises are short bursts of intense activity followed by rest periods or low-intensity exercise. For example, sprint for 30 seconds, followed by a minute of walking, repeating this cycle for 15-20 minutes. This type of exercise has improved cardiovascular health, increased metabolic rate, and enhanced HRV. Include HIIT sessions two to three times a week for optimal results.

To create a guided physical activity routine:

1. Start with a warm-up. Spend five minutes doing light cardio exercises like marching in place or gentle jogging to increase blood flow and prepare your muscles.
2. Next, move to the main activities. Combine aerobics, strength training, and flexibility exercises in a balanced routine. For example, you might start with 10 minutes of jogging, 15 minutes of weight lifting, and 10 minutes of yoga.
3. End with a cool-down, stretching all major muscle groups to improve flexibility and prevent injury.

CHAPTER 6

Staying motivated and consistent with your physical activity routine is crucial for long-term success. Set realistic and achievable goals to keep yourself on track. For instance, try to walk 10,000 steps a day or complete three strength training sessions a week. Finding a workout buddy or joining the right gym can provide accountability and support. Keep a workout journal to log your progress and celebrate your achievements. Using fitness apps can help you stay organized and motivated. Reward yourself for consistency and progress, whether it's a relaxing bath after a workout or a new piece of exercise equipment.

Engaging in regular physical activity supports weight loss and enhances your overall physical and mental health. Exercise becomes vital to your journey toward better health by improving vagal tone, reducing stress, and promoting relaxation.

INTEGRATING VAGUS NERVE EXERCISES INTO A SUSTAINABLE WEIGHT LOSS PLAN

Integrating vagus nerve exercises into your plan can make all the difference. This isn't about quick fixes or crash diets. It's about creating a balanced life that supports long-term health. Combining diet, exercise, and stress management is crucial. You need to address not just what you eat and how much you move but also your emotional and psychological well-being. Focus on these elements to create a sustainable lifestyle that promotes weight loss and overall health.

Start by setting realistic and achievable goals. Aim for modest, attainable milestones rather than drastic changes. For example, losing one to two pounds per week is a healthy and sustainable goal. Next, develop a balanced, nutrient-rich diet plan. Include food like fruits, vegetables, lean proteins, and whole grains in your diet. Avoid processed foods and sugary drinks. Establish a regular physical activity routine that includes a mix of aerobic, strength, and flexibility exercises. This combination ensures you burn calories, build muscle, and stay flexible.

Incorporate stress management techniques to support your plan. Mindfulness and meditation can be powerful tools. These exercises can help calm your mind and reduce the stress linked to emotional eating. Spend a few minutes each day meditating or simply being mindful. Focus on your breath, clear your mind, and let go of stress.

Maintaining your weight loss plan requires practical strategies. Note what you eat, how much you exercise, and how you feel. This helps you stay accountable and track your progress. Seek support from friends, family, or a weight loss group. Sharing your journey with others provides encouragement and motivation. Stay flexible and make adjustments as needed. Life happens, and sometimes you'll need to adapt your plan. That's okay. It's okay to take a break, but the key is to always get back on track when you can.

Celebrating milestones and progress is also essential. Reward yourself for hitting your goals. These rewards can keep you focused on your long-term goals. Real-life success stories can be very inspiring. Take, for instance, Lisa, who successfully integrated vagus nerve exercises into her weight loss plan. She started with small, realistic goals, developed a balanced diet, and established a regular exercise routine. By incorporating mindfulness and meditation, Lisa managed her stress and avoided emotional eating. Over time, she achieved sustainable weight loss and improved her overall well-being.

Integrating vagus nerve exercises into your weight loss plan can lead to sustainable, long-term results. Combining diet, exercise, and stress management creates a focused approach that addresses all aspects of your health. Remember, it's not about quick fixes but about making lasting lifestyle changes.

CHAPTER 6

Weight Loss
Vagus Nerve Exercises
Video Guide

CHAPTER 7
YOGA AND PHYSICAL EXERCISES

RESTORATIVE YOGA: GENTLE POSES FOR VAGUS NERVE STIMULATION

Restorative yoga is a practice that promotes deep relaxation and rejuvenation through gentle stretches and supported poses. Unlike other vigorous forms of yoga, restorative yoga focuses on activating the parasympathetic nervous system, which is responsible for the "rest and digest" functions of the body. By encouraging a state of calm and relaxation, restorative yoga helps reduce stress and anxiety, making it an effective tool for enhancing vagal tone.

The key to restorative yoga is using props such as bolsters, blankets, and blocks to support the body in various poses. This support allows you to hold poses for extended periods without strain, promoting deep stretching and relaxation. By gently stimulating the vagus nerve, these poses can help regulate heart rate and improve digestion.

One of the foundational poses in restorative yoga is the **Supported Child's Pose (Balasana):**

1. Kneel down with your big toes touching and your knees spread wide apart.
2. Sit back on your heels and place a bolster lengthwise in front of you.
3. Lean forward, resting your torso on the bolster, and turn your head to one side.
4. Extend your arms forward or let them rest alongside the bolster.
5. Hold this pose for several minutes, allowing your body to relax completely.

The gentle pressure on your abdomen and the support of the bolster help stimulate the vagus nerve and promote a sense of calm.

Another highly effective pose is the **Legs-Up-the-Wall Pose (Viparita Karani)**. This pose is ideal for reducing stress and improving circulation:

1. Sit down sideways against a wall with your knees bent and feet on the floor.
2. Slowly lie back and swing your legs up the wall, forming an L-shape with your body.
3. Place a folded blanket or cushion below your hips for added support.
4. Dangle your arms at your sides with your palms facing up.
5. Close your eyes & focus on your breath.
6. Hold this pose for 5 to 15 minutes, allowing the gentle inversion to calm your nervous system and stimulate the vagus nerve.

The **Reclining Bound Angle Pose (Supta Baddha Konasana)** is another restorative favorite that opens the chest and hips while promoting relaxation. To perform this pose:

CHAPTER 7

1. Lie on your back with a bolster or folded blanket under your spine.
2. Bend your knees and keep the soles of your feet together
3. Let your knees fall open to the sides.
4. Use blocks or additional blankets under your knees for support.
5. Extend your arms out to the sides & keep your palms facing up.
6. Close your eyes, breathe deeply & hold the pose for several minutes.

This gentle stretch helps open the chest and stimulate the vagus nerve, promoting relaxation.

Props and modifications are essential in restorative yoga to ensure comfort and effectiveness. Using bolsters, blankets, and blocks can help you find the perfect alignment and support for each pose. For example, placing cushions under your knees in the Reclining Bound Angle Pose can alleviate discomfort if you have tight hips. Similarly, a folded blanket under your head in the Supported Child's Pose can provide additional support for your neck. These modifications make restorative yoga accessible to individuals of all flexibility levels, ensuring everyone can benefit from the practice.

Real-life testimonials highlight the profound impact of restorative yoga on mental and physical well-being. Jessica, a busy professional, shares how incorporating these gentle poses into her evening routine helped her reduce chronic stress and improve sleep quality. She found that the deep relaxation promoted by restorative yoga allowed her to release tension accumulated throughout the day, leading to more restful nights. Another practitioner, Tom, discovered that restorative yoga enhanced his emotional balance and overall sense of calm. By regularly practicing poses like Supported Child's Pose and Legs-Up-the-Wall, he experienced a significant reduction in anxiety and stress.

Restorative yoga offers a simple yet powerful way to stimulate the vagus nerve. By focusing on gentle stretches and deep relaxation, this practice activates the parasympathetic nervous system, decreasing stress and anxiety. Through props and modifications, restorative yoga is accessible to individuals of all flexibility levels, ensuring everyone can experience its benefits. As you add these poses into your daily routine, you may find yourself experiencing a profound sense of peace and balance, much like Martha, Jessica, and Tom.

SUN SALUTATIONS: ENERGIZING YOUR VAGUS NERVE

Imagine standing at the start of your day, feeling the warmth of the morning sun on your skin. Sun Salutations, or Surya Namaskara, is a dynamic sequence of yoga poses that honor the sun and invigorate the body and mind. This ancient practice energizes you and activates the vagus nerve, which plays a crucial role in maintaining balance within the body. By flowing through these poses, you engage in a form of moving meditation that improves cardiovascular health.

To start, stand tall in **Mountain Pose (Tadasana)**:

1. Ground your feet firmly into the floor, feeling the connection to the earth.
2. Your arms should rest by your sides, palms facing forward.
3. Take a deep breath, lift your arms overhead, and reach toward the sky.

This pose establishes a stable foundation, preparing you for the sequence ahead.

Next, transition into the **Forward Fold (Uttanasana)**:

1. Exhale as you hinge at the hips, bringing your torso down towards your thighs.
2. Allow your hands to rest on the floor or grasp the back of your legs.
3. Feel the stretch in your hamstrings & the release of tension in your back.

This pose encourages a calm mind, reducing stress and anxiety.

From the **Forward Fold**, move into the **Plank Pose (Phalakasana)**:

1. Place your hands on the floor, step your feet back, and align your body into a straight line from head to heels.
2. Engage your core, keep your shoulders over your wrists, and maintain a steady breath.

Plank Pose builds strength and stability, which is crucial for enhancing overall body function.

Transition smoothly into **Upward-Facing Dog (Urdhva Mukha Svanasana)**:

1. Lower your hips towards the floor.
2. Keep your legs extended and the tops of the feet pressing into the mat.
3. Straighten your arms, raise your chest, and look slightly upward.

This backbend opens the chest and activates the vagus nerve, promoting a sense of openness and vitality.

Next, flow into **Downward-Facing Dog (Adho Mukha Svanasana)**:

1. Lift your hips towards the sky.
2. Form an inverted V shape with your body.

3. Press your hands firmly into the mat & spread your fingers wide.
4. Lengthen your spine and let your heels drift towards the floor.
5. Return to Mountain Pose by stepping forward and rising up, completing the sequence.

This pose calms the mind, stretches the entire body, and enhances circulation.

With consistent practice, Sun Salutations can significantly improve your health. The rhythmic movement and mindful breathing increase energy levels, making you feel more alert and alive. Regular practice also improves flexibility and strength, reducing the risk of injuries and enhancing physical resilience. Additionally, the meditative aspect enhances mental clarity, allowing you to focus better and manage stress more effectively.

For beginners, adapting the practice to your comfort level is essential. Feel free to bend your knees slightly in Forward Fold to ease the stretch on your hamstrings. In Plank Pose, you can lower your knees to the floor if holding a full plank is challenging. For Upward-Facing Dog, you might start with Cobra Pose, keeping your elbows bent and lifting only your chest. These modifications ensure that you can practice safely and build strength gradually.

Experienced yogis can explore advanced variations to deepen their practice. To increase the intensity, you might add a Chaturanga Dandasana (Low Plank) between the Plank and Upward-Facing Dog. Holding each pose for a few extra breaths can also enhance the challenge, building greater endurance and focus.

Sun Salutations provide a holistic approach to invigorating your body and mind. By incorporating these sequences into your daily routine, you tap into the power of the vagus nerve, promoting relaxation and resilience. Whether you're a beginner finding your way or an advanced practitioner seeking to deepen your experience, Sun Salutations offer a versatile and impactful practice.

GENTLE STRETCHING ROUTINES: DAILY PRACTICES

Picture starting your day with a gentle stretch, feeling the stiffness melt away as you ease into the morning. Gentle stretching can significantly enhance the health of your vagus nerve, promoting relaxation and reducing muscle tension. When you stretch, you help improve circulation, delivering oxygen and nutrients to your tissues and muscles. This not only enhances flexibility but also supports overall well-being. Stretching engages the parasympathetic nervous system, aiding in the reduction of stress and anxiety and nurturing a feeling of tranquility and equilibrium in your everyday life. A daily stretching routine can work wonders for your body and mind.

Begin with **Neck Stretches**:

1. Sit or stand comfortably, keeping your spine straight.
2. Tilt your head to the right & bring your ear towards your shoulder.
3. Hold this position for a few breaths, feeling the stretch along the left side of your neck.
4. Slowly return to the center and repeat on the other side.

Next, move on to **Shoulder Rolls**:

1. Sit or stand with your arms dangling by your sides.
2. Inhale as you lift your shoulders toward your ears.
3. Exhale as you roll them back and down.
4. Repeat this motion a few times to release shoulder and upper back tension.

Incorporate the **Seated Forward Bend (Paschimottanasana)** into your routine for a deeper stretch:

1. Sit down on the floor with your legs stretched towards the front.
2. Inhale as you lengthen your spine.
3. Exhale as you hinge at your hips & bring your hands towards your feet.
4. Allow your torso to bend over your legs & keep your back straight.
5. Hold this pose for several breaths, feeling the stretch along your hamstrings and lower back.

The gentle forward fold helps calm the mind and stimulate the vagus nerve.

The **Cat-Cow Pose (Marjaryasana-Bitilasana)** is another excellent addition to your stretching routine:

1. Begin on your hands and knees in a tabletop position.
2. As you inhale, lower your stomach towards the mat.
3. Lift your head and tailbone, and arch your back (Cow Pose).
4. On the exhale, round your spine, tuck your chin towards your chest, and bring your belly button towards your spine (Cat Pose).
5. Flow between these two positions with each breath, allowing your spine to move fluidly.

This dynamic stretch increases spinal flexibility, reduces tension, and stimulates the vagus nerve.

Regular stretching offers numerous benefits beyond enhanced vagal tone. It decreases the risk of injury by improving your flexibility, making everyday tasks and physical exercises safer.

Stretching also improves posture and alignment, helping to alleviate discomfort caused by poor posture. Additionally, stretching promotes relaxation and stress relief, providing a moment of mindfulness and self-care in your day. Studies have demonstrated that stretching activates the parasympathetic nervous system, reducing stress and anxiety levels. Incorporating gentle stretching into your daily life can profoundly impact your physical and mental health.

BALANCING POSES: ENHANCING VAGAL TONE

Balancing poses in yoga offer a unique blend of physical and mental benefits, making them an important part of any practice. These poses require focus and concentration, as you must stabilize your body and maintain equilibrium. This mental engagement helps improve cognitive functions, enhancing attention and clarity. Additionally, balancing poses increase body awareness and coordination, which are crucial for daily activities and overall physical health. By engaging the core and stabilizing muscles, you activate the parasympathetic nervous system. This combination of benefits makes balancing poses an effective way to enhance vagal tone.

One of the foundational balancing poses is **Tree Pose (Vrksasana)**:

1. Begin by standing up with your feet hip-width apart.
2. Place your weight onto your left foot and ground it firmly into the floor.
3. Slowly lift your right foot and place it on your inner left thigh or calf while avoiding the knee.
4. Bring your hands to your heart center in a prayer position or extend them overhead like branches.
5. Focus on a fixed point in front of you to help you maintain balance.
6. Hold the pose for several breaths.
7. Switch sides.

Tree Pose improves stability and strengthens the legs while calming the mind.

Warrior III (Virabhadrasana III) is another powerful balancing pose that engages the entire body:

1. Start in a standing position with your feet together.
2. Place your weight onto your right foot and extend your arms overhead.
3. Hinge at your hips, lifting your left leg behind you while keeping it straight. Your body should form a straight line from fingertips to toes.
4. Focus on a point in front of you to help you maintain balance.
5. Hold the pose for several breaths.
6. Switch sides.

Warrior III enhances coordination and strengthens the core, legs, and back, making it an excellent pose for improving vagal tone.

Eagle Pose (Garudasana) offers a unique challenge by requiring you to balance while twisting your limbs:

1. Begin by standing tall with your feet together.
2. Fold your knees slightly and lift your right foot, wrapping it around your left leg.
3. Cross your left arm over your right, bringing your palms together if possible.
4. Sink deeper into your standing leg and focus on a fixed point.
5. Hold the pose for several breaths.
6. Switch sides.

Eagle Pose enhances body awareness, improves focus, and

strengthens the legs and arms. The twisting motion also helps stimulate the vagus nerve, promoting relaxation.

Half Moon Pose (Ardha Chandrasana) combines balance, strength, and flexibility:

1. Begin in a standing position with your feet together.
2. Bring your right foot back and bend your left knee slightly.
3. Place your left hand on the floor or a block in front of your left foot.
4. Lift your right leg parallel to the floor & extend your right arm towards the ceiling.
5. Your body should form a straight line from your right heel to your right hand.
6. Focus on a fixed point to help you maintain balance.
7. Hold the pose for a few breaths.
8. Switch sides.

Half Moon Pose improves stability, strengthens the legs and core, and enhances mental clarity.

Balance is critical in our daily lives, influencing everything from walking to navigating uneven surfaces. Balancing poses improve stability and coordination, reducing the risk of falls and injuries. They also enhance mental clarity and focus, allowing you to stay present and engaged in your activities. Additionally, balancing poses promote emotional regulation, helping you manage stress and anxiety more effectively.

When practicing balancing poses, it's important to use props for support if needed. Placing a block or chair nearby can provide extra stability, especially for beginners. Practicing near a wall can also offer support, allowing you to focus on alignment without fear of falling. Focusing on a fixed point, or drishti, helps maintain balance by providing a visual anchor. Regular practice of balancing poses can significantly improve your stability and coordination.

Adding balancing poses into your yoga practice can significantly enhance vagal tone and promote overall health. These poses improve focus, body awareness, and coordination while activating the parasympathetic nervous system. Whether you are a beginner or an experienced yogi, balancing poses offer a versatile and effective way to enhance your practice and well-being.

CHAPTER 7

Yoga
Vagus Nerve Exercises
Video Guide

CHAPTER 8
DEEP SLEEP STRATEGIES

BEDTIME BREATHING EXERCISES FOR BETTER SLEEP

Bedtime breathing exercises are crucial for preparing your body and mind for sleep. These methods function by stimulating the parasympathetic nervous system, which aids in relaxing your body after a demanding day. When this system is activated, your heart rate slows, and your blood pressure lowers, fostering a sense of calm. This response is crucial for alleviating stress and anxiety, both of which often contribute to sleep issues. As your body becomes more at ease, you're more inclined to drift off quickly and experience a restful, uninterrupted sleep.

One effective technique to try is the **4-7-8 Breathing** method:

1. Sit or lay down in a comfortable position.
2. Close your eyes and let your body relax.
3. Inhale through your nose for four seconds.
4. Hold your breath for seven seconds.
5. Exhale through your mouth for eight seconds.

6. Repeat this cycle four times initially.
7. Gradually increasing as you become more comfortable with the practice.

This method helps to regulate your breathing, slow your heart rate, and calm your nervous system, making it easier to drift off to sleep.

Another beneficial technique is **Alternate Nostril Breathing**, also known as **Nadi Shodhana**:

1. Sit comfortably with a straight spine.
2. Close your right nostril with your right thumb and inhale through your left nostril.
3. Close your left nostril & exhale through your right nostril.
4. Inhale through your right nostril, close it & exhale through your left nostril.
5. Repeat this pattern for several minutes.

This practice balances your autonomic nervous system, enhances mental clarity, and reduces stress, setting the stage for a restful night.

Pursed-Lip Breathing is another simple yet effective method:

1. Begin by sitting or lying down comfortably.
2. Inhale through your nose for two seconds.
3. Purse your lips as if you're about to blow out a candle.
4. Exhale slowly for four seconds.

This technique helps to slow your breathing, reduce shortness of breath, and promote relaxation. Practicing pursed-lip breathing before bed can help calm your mind and body, preparing you for a peaceful night's sleep.

CHAPTER 8

Guided Bedtime Breathing Practice

To enhance your **Bedtime Breathing** exercises:

1. Create a calming environment.
2. Find a dark, quiet space where you can lie down comfortably.
3. Use calming background music or nature sounds to set a peaceful atmosphere. Essential oils like lavender can also help you relax.

Begin with the 4-7-8 Breathing method, followed by Alternate Nostril Breathing, Deep Diaphragmatic Breathing, and Pursed-Lip Breathing. Spend about five minutes on each technique. Focus on the timing of your inhales, holds, and exhales, ensuring you breathe slowly and deeply. Practicing these exercises regularly can help you develop a consistent bedtime routine, leading to better sleep quality.

THE BENEFITS OF RESTORATIVE YOGA FOR INSOMNIA

Restorative yoga is a gentle practice that can be incredibly effective for alleviating insomnia. By stimulating the vagus nerve, restorative yoga activates the parasympathetic nervous system. This activation helps to calm your body, reducing muscle tension and stress. When the parasympathetic system is engaged, your body naturally shifts into a state of deep relaxation. This state is crucial for improving sleep onset and quality. The gentle, sustained postures in restorative yoga promote a sense of calmness, making it easier for you to transition from the busyness of the day to a restful night.

One of the most impactful restorative yoga poses is the **Legs-Up-the-Wall Pose (Viparita Karani)**. To practice this pose:

1. Sit sideways against a wall.
2. Extend your legs along the floor.
3. Lay back and swing your legs up the wall, forming an L-shape with your body.
4. Your hips should be close to the wall, and your arms can rest comfortably at your sides.
5. Hold this position for five to fifteen minutes.

This gentle inversion encourages blood flow away from the legs. It helps to calm the nervous system, bringing relaxation and preparing your body for sleep.

Another effective pose is the **Supported Child's Pose (Balasana)**:

1. Start by kneeling on the floor with your big toes touching & knees spread wide.
2. Sit on your heels & extend your arms in front of you.
3. Lower your torso between your thighs.
4. Place a bolster or a rolled blanket under your torso for support, allowing your forehead to rest on the prop.
5. Hold this pose for five to ten minutes.

The Supported Child's Pose helps release tension in the back and shoulders, promoting a sense of safety and calmness, which is conducive to sleep.

The **Reclining Bound Angle Pose (Supta Baddha Konasana)** is another excellent posture for improving sleep:

1. Lie on your back and bring the soles of your feet together, letting your knees fall open to the sides.
2. Place a bolster or pillows under your knees for support.
3. Rest your arms at your sides with palms facing up.
4. Hold this position for five to ten minutes.

CHAPTER 8

This pose will help open up the hips and chest, encouraging deep breathing and relaxation.

Supported Bridge Pose (Setu Bandhasana) is also beneficial:

1. Lie on your back with your knees bent & feet flat on the floor, hip-width apart.
2. Use a block or bolster under your sacrum for support, lifting your hips off the ground.
3. Rest your arms at your sides.
4. Hold this pose for five to ten minutes.

Supported Bridge Pose helps to stretch the chest, neck, and spine, promoting relaxation and reducing stress.

Guided Restorative Yoga Routine:

Begin your restorative yoga session with a few warm-up exercises like gentle neck rolls or shoulder shrugs to loosen up. Move into the Legs-Up-the-Wall Pose, holding for five to fifteen minutes, focusing on your breath. Transition to Supported Child's Pose, holding for five to ten minutes, allowing your body to relax deeply. Move into Reclining Bound Angle Pose, staying for five to ten minutes, and then finish with Supported Bridge Pose for another five to ten minutes. Conclude with a brief relaxation period, lying flat on your back with eyes closed, breathing deeply.

To practice safely, always listen to your body's signals. Avoid any pose that causes pain or discomfort. Use props like bolsters, blankets, and blocks to support your body and enhance comfort. Practicing in a dark, quiet environment can further enhance the calming effects of restorative yoga, helping you prepare for a restful night's sleep.

GUIDED IMAGERY FOR RELAXING THE MIND AND BODY

Imagine this: after a long day filled with endless tasks and responsibilities, you finally lie down in bed, but your mind refuses to quiet down. This is where guided imagery can make a significant difference. Guided imagery is a relaxation practice that involves visualizing calming and peaceful scenes to help reduce stress and anxiety. By engaging your mind in positive and soothing images, you stimulate the vagus nerve, promoting relaxation and calmness. This practice helps to enhance mental focus and emotional stability, making it easier for you to fall asleep and enjoy a restful night.

To get started with **Guided Imagery**:

1. Consider picturing a serene, calming location.
2. Close your eyes and imagine a peaceful place, such as a quiet beach with gentle waves lapping at the shore or a lush forest with birds chirping and leaves flowing with the breeze.
3. Focus on the details: the colors, sounds, and scents.

This mental escape can help you shift your focus away from stressors and nurture a sense of tranquility.

Another effective technique is **Body Scanning Imagery**:

1. Begin by lying down in a comfortable position and closing your eyes.
2. Visualize each part of your body, starting from your toes and moving up to your head.
3. Imagine a warm, soothing light washing over each area, releasing tension and promoting relaxation.

Color Imagery is another powerful method:

1. Close your eyes and imagine a soothing color, such as blue or green, flowing through your body with each breath.
2. Visualize this color as a warm, healing light that calms your mind and body, easing you into a state of deep relaxation.

Nature Imagery can also be incredibly effective:

1. Picture yourself in a natural setting that you find calming, such as a meadow filled with wildflowers, a mountain stream with crystal-clear water, or a starlit night sky.

Engaging your senses in this way can help lower stress levels and help your body fall asleep.

Guided Imagery Session for Sleep

1. Start by finding a comfortable, lying-down position in a quiet environment.
2. Begin with a few minutes of deep breathing to relax your body and mind.
3. Close your eyes and choose one of the imagery techniques mentioned earlier.

For example, if you choose peaceful place imagery, visualize your serene location in vivid detail. Focus on the sights, sounds, and scents, allowing yourself to immerse in the scene fully. Spend about 10-15 minutes on this exercise, then gradually bring your awareness back to the present moment. Take a few more deep breaths before opening your eyes and preparing for sleep. For guided imagery to be most effective, practice it regularly. Consistency helps reinforce the relaxation response and makes it easier for you to transition into sleep.

If staying focused during guided imagery is difficult, consider utilizing audio recordings or apps designed for guided imagery sessions. Pairing this practice with relaxation methods like deep breathing or meditation can enhance its impact. Incorporating guided imagery into your nightly routine can be a valuable tool for managing stress, fostering relaxation, and improving your sleep.

CREATING A SLEEP-INDUCING EVENING ROUTINE

Developing an evening routine is crucial for preparing your body and mind for sleep. Establishing a regular sleep routine aids in balancing your internal clock, which simplifies the process of falling asleep and waking up at the same time every day.

Consistency reinforces your body's natural sleep-wake cycle, promoting better sleep quality. Reducing exposure to blue light and stimulating activities at least an hour before bed is equally important. Blue light from screens can hurt melatonin production, the hormone that regulates sleep. By limiting screen time and practicing calming activities, you create an environment conducive to sleep. This approach not only helps you relax but also improves sleep onset, helping you fall asleep faster and enjoy a more restful night.

Incorporating specific elements into your evening routine can make a significant difference. Start by setting a regular sleep and wake-up time. Consistency is vital, even on weekends. Try out relaxing activities such as reading a book, journaling your thoughts, or listening to chill music. These activities can help you unwind and signal to your body that it's time to prepare for sleep. Limiting screen time is essential; consider turning off your phone at least an hour before bed. Instead, create a calming bedtime environment with dim lighting and comfortable bedding. This setting enhances the relaxation needed for a good night's sleep.

CHAPTER 8

To create an effective evening routine, begin with mind-body relaxation techniques like deep breathing or meditation. These exercises help calm your nervous system and prepare your body for rest. Next, engage in calming activities. Reading a book can be a soothing way to end the day, while journaling allows you to clear your mind and set aside any lingering worries. Afterward, prepare your bedroom for sleep. Turn off the lights, adjust the room temperature to your ideal level, and ensure your bedding is inviting. Establish a consistent bedtime ritual, such as drinking a cup of herbal tea or taking a warm bath. These rituals signal to your body that it's time to wind down.

Maintaining a sleep-inducing evening routine requires patience and consistency. Start by keeping a sleep journal to track your progress and make necessary adjustments. Note any patterns or activities that seem to improve or disrupt your sleep. Be patient with yourself as you establish this new routine. It may take some time to see significant changes, but consistency is key. Make gradual changes to your routine to avoid disrupting your sleep patterns. If you live with family or roommates, seek their support in maintaining a peaceful environment. Encourage them to respect your bedtime routine and create a quiet atmosphere conducive to sleep.

Creating a sleep-inducing evening routine can transform your sleep quality by helping you relax and manage stress. By adding these practices to your nightly routine, you can stimulate the vagus nerve and prepare your body for a restful night. Establishing consistency, reducing blue light exposure, and engaging in calming activities are vital steps to improving your sleep. As you adopt these practices, you'll find that a well-structured evening routine can significantly affect your sleep quality and daily life.

Sleep Disorders
Vagus Nerve Exercises Video Guide

CHAPTER 9
COLD EXPOSURE TECHNIQUES

COLD SHOWERS: A BEGINNER'S GUIDE

Though seemingly simple, cold showers hold immense potential for stimulating the vagus nerve. When you step into a cold shower, your body undergoes a series of physiological responses that activate the parasympathetic nervous system. This activation produces a state of calm and relaxation, counteracting the body's stress response. Additionally, cold showers help reduce inflammation, a common culprit behind chronic pain and various health issues. Cold exposure can effectively decrease inflammation by constricting blood vessels and decreasing blood flow to inflamed areas. But the benefits don't stop there. Cold showers also enhance mental clarity and focus by increasing blood flow to the brain. This boost in circulation can help you feel more alert and energized. Moreover, the invigorating nature of cold water can improve mood and energy levels, leaving you feeling refreshed and motivated.

To add **Cold Showers** into your routine, it's essential to ease into the practice gradually:

1. Begin with your usual warm shower to relax your muscles and prepare your body.
2. Once you're comfortable, slowly reduce the temperature until the water is cold.
3. At first, aim to spend about 30 seconds under the cold water.
4. As you become more accustomed to the sensation, gradually increase the duration to 2-3 minutes.

This incremental approach helps your body get used to the cold, minimizing discomfort. Maintaining comfort and safety during cold showers is crucial. Ensure the water isn't too cold initially, and always listen to your body's signals. If you start feeling too uncomfortable or chilled, it's perfectly okay to revert to warmer water and try again another time. The goal is to make cold showers a sustainable part of your routine, not a source of stress.

The body's response to cold showers involves a fascinating series of physiological reactions. Initially, the cold water triggers a shock response, causing your body to gasp and your heart rate to spike. This reaction is part of the body's survival mechanism. However, with continued exposure, your body begins to adapt. The shock response diminishes, and you start to experience the benefits. One benefit is the release of endorphins and adrenaline. These feel-good hormones elevate your mood and provide a natural energy boost. Cold showers also improve circulation by constricting and dilating blood vessels, promoting better blood flow throughout the body. This process enhances cardiovascular health and increases metabolic rate, aiding in weight regulation and overall vitality.

Cold showers offer a simple yet powerful way to stimulate your vagus nerve and enhance your overall health. By gradually incorporating them into your routine, you can experience reduced inflammation, enhanced mental clarity, improved mood, and increased energy levels. The initial discomfort is a small price to pay for the profound benefits that await. So why not take the plunge and see how cold showers can transform your health?

ICE BATHS: STEP-BY-STEP INSTRUCTIONS

Imagine stepping into a tub filled with icy water and feeling the cold envelop you. This is the essence of an ice bath, a more intense form of cold exposure that offers profound health benefits. When you immerse yourself in an ice bath, you significantly enhance vagal tone, activating the parasympathetic nervous system. This activation helps your body enter a state of rest and recovery, contrasting sharply with the stress-induced fight-or-flight mode. Ice baths also substantially reduce muscle soreness and inflammation, making them a favored recovery method among athletes. The cold water constricts blood vessels to reduce blood flow to muscles and inflamed areas, which helps in quicker recovery from physical exertion. Beyond physical benefits, ice baths can improve mental resilience and toughness. The sheer act of enduring the cold builds mental fortitude, teaching you to remain calm under stress. Enhanced vagal tone, reduced muscle soreness, accelerated recovery, and improved mental toughness make ice baths a valuable addition to your wellness routine.

You'll need some essential equipment to start incorporating **Ice Baths** into your routine:

- Sturdy tub
- Plenty of ice
- Thermometer

To get started:

1. Begin by filling the tub with cold water before gradually adding ice.

2. Chill the water to a temperature between 50-59°F (10-15°C) for best results.
3. Begin with 5-10 minutes, gradually increasing as your body adapts to the cold.

Safety is paramount, so keep a warm towel or blanket nearby to wrap yourself in immediately after exiting the ice bath. Keeping track of your body temperature is crucial to avoid hypothermia. Always listen to your body; if you feel too uncomfortable or chilled, it's okay to cut the session short and try again another time. The goal is to make this practice sustainable and beneficial, not a source of stress.

The physiological responses to ice baths are fascinating and multifaceted. When you first enter the icy water, your body undergoes vasoconstriction, where blood vessels constrict to preserve heat. This initial response is followed by vasodilation once you exit the bath, where blood vessels expand, promoting blood flow and healing. This process helps reduce inflammation markers in the body, aiding quicker recovery from physical exertion. Additionally, cold exposure activates the release of endorphins and adrenaline, hormones that elevate your mood and provide a natural energy boost. The combination of these physiological responses enhances overall well-being, making ice baths a powerful tool for both physical and mental health.

Consider the experience of athletes who regularly incorporate ice baths into their recovery routines. Take John, a marathon runner, who found that ice baths significantly reduced his muscle soreness after long runs. This allowed him to train more consistently without the prolonged recovery periods needed before. Another example is Lisa, a fitness enthusiast, who noticed an improvement in her mental resilience. Enduring the cold water helped her develop a stronger mindset, enabling her to handle stress more effectively in her daily life. Scientific research supports these benefits. A study from the Mayo Clinic highlights how cold-water immersion can reduce inflammation and soreness, aiding in physical performance recovery. The study emphasizes the role of ice baths in enhancing recovery by promoting rapid constriction and subsequent dilation of blood vessels, which helps flush out metabolic waste and reduce muscle damage.

Ice baths offer a robust method to stimulate the vagus nerve and reap significant health benefits. You can add this powerful technique into your wellness routine by following the steps for safe practice. The physiological responses, from vasoconstriction to the release of endorphins, provide a comprehensive approach to enhancing physical and mental resilience.

CRYOTHERAPY: AN OVERVIEW AND HOW TO ACCESS IT

Cryotherapy, a technique that exposes the body to extreme cold, offers a unique way to enhance health. Unlike cold showers or ice baths, cryotherapy often involves whole-body exposure or targeted, localized treatment. Whole-body cryotherapy (WBC) involves stepping into a chamber cooled to extremely low temperatures, typically between -200°F and -300°F, for a brief period, usually 2-3 minutes. On the other hand, localized cryotherapy targets specific areas using devices like cryogenic wands or ice packs.

The benefits of cryotherapy are significant and multifaceted. One of the primary advantages is its ability to reduce inflammation and alleviate pain. This is particularly helpful for people suffering from chronic pain conditions or recovering from injuries. Cryotherapy also enhances vagal tone, promoting relaxation by activating the parasympathetic nervous system. This can help reduce stress. Additionally, cryotherapy has been shown to improve skin health and boost collagen production, leading to a more youthful appearance. The cold exposure helps tighten pores, reduce acne, and improve skin elasticity.

When preparing for a cryotherapy session, knowing what to expect is essential. Before entering the cryotherapy chamber, you will be given protective gear (gloves, socks, and sometimes a headband to protect sensitive areas from frostbite). It's recommended to wear minimal clothing, usually just undergarments, as this allows maximum exposure to the cold air. The session itself is brief but intense, lasting only 2-3 minutes. During this time, the chamber is cooled to temperatures as low as -300°F. After the session, warming up is crucial. Most cryotherapy centers provide warm blankets or heated rooms to help your body adjust back to normal temperatures. Hydration is also vital, as the cold exposure can be dehydrating.

Accessing cryotherapy services has become increasingly convenient as more centers and spas offer this treatment. You can find cryotherapy facilities in many urban areas, often within wellness centers or specialized cryotherapy clinics. It's advisable to check reviews and ensure the center follows safety protocols. Cost considerations vary, with single sessions typically costing $40 to $100. Some centers offer packages or memberships that can reduce the per-session cost. Insurance coverage for cryotherapy is uncommon, so it's best to check with your provider. For those interested in home treatments, cryotherapy devices are available for purchase. While these are less intense than professional sessions, they offer a convenient alternative. Home devices can target specific areas and are generally more affordable in the long run, though they require proper usage to ensure safety.

Whether whole-body or localized, cryotherapy offers a powerful means to enhance health. You can make the most of this innovative treatment by understanding the process, preparing adequately, and knowing where to access services. The benefits, supported by personal testimonials and scientific research, make cryotherapy a valuable addition to your wellness routine.

COMBINING COLD EXPOSURE WITH BREATHING TECHNIQUES

Combining cold exposure with specific breathing techniques can amplify the benefits of both practices, creating a powerful approach to enhancing overall health. Combining these methods significantly improves vagal tone and activates the parasympathetic nervous system more effectively. This combination helps your body shift from a state of stress to one of relaxation, improving your ability to handle daily pressures easily. The synergy between cold exposure and breathing exercises also boosts oxygen uptake and circulation, leading to better physical performance and quicker recovery times. Additionally, these practices work together to reduce inflammation, which is crucial for managing chronic pain.

One of the most well-known methods that integrate deep breathing with cold exposure is the **Wim Hof Method**. This technique involves a series of powerful inhalations and relaxed exhalations, followed by breath holds. To practice it:

1. Start by sitting comfortably, taking 30 deep breaths, inhaling fully, and letting the breath go without forcing the exhale.
2. After the last breath, hold your breath for as long as you can comfortably manage, then take a deep breath in and hold it for 15 seconds before letting go.
3. Repeat this cycle three times. Once you've completed the breathing exercises, you can proceed with cold exposure, such as an ice bath or cold shower.

This method prepares your body for the cold and enhances mental focus and resilience.

Another effective technique is **Box Breathing**, which calms the mind and body before and during cold exposure:

1. Sit comfortably and breathe in for four seconds.
2. Hold your breath for four seconds.
3. Exhale for four seconds.
4. Hold your breath again for four seconds.
5. Repeat this cycle for several minutes.

This method helps regulate your breathing, making the cold exposure more manageable and less shocking to the system. By calming your mind and body, you prepare yourself to face the cold with a sense of calm and control, enhancing the overall benefits of the practice.

The physiological and psychological benefits of combining cold exposure with these breathing techniques are profound. Improved mental clarity and focus are among the most noticeable effects. The increased oxygen uptake from deep breathing, combined with the invigorating nature of cold exposure, leaves you feeling alert and mentally sharp. Additionally, these practices significantly reduce anxiety and stress levels. Activating the parasympathetic nervous system through cold exposure and controlled breathing promotes a state of relaxation and calmness, helping you handle stress more effectively. Improved physical resilience and quicker recovery times are also notable benefits. The anti-inflammatory effects of cold exposure, coupled with the enhanced oxygenation from deep breathing, aid in faster recovery from physical exertion and reduce muscle soreness.

Consider the experience of athletes who have adopted this combined approach. Take Mike, a triathlete, who found that inte-

CHAPTER 9

grating the Wim Hof Method with ice baths significantly improved his endurance and recovery. He reported feeling more energized during training sessions and experienced quicker recovery times, allowing him to train more consistently.

By combining cold exposure with specific breathing techniques, you can unlock a powerful approach to enhancing your overall health. These practices work together to boost vagal tone, reduce stress, improve mental clarity, and accelerate recovery. The synergy between cold exposure and controlled breathing offers a comprehensive method for better physical and psychological well-being. So, whether you're an athlete looking to improve performance or someone seeking to enhance overall health, this combined approach holds immense potential for transformative benefits.

Cold Exposure
Vagus Nerve Exercises Video Guide

CHAPTER 10
DIET AND LIFESTYLE CHANGES

ANTI-INFLAMMATORY DIET: FOODS TO INCLUDE

Reducing inflammation is crucial for maintaining optimal vagal tone and overall health. Chronic inflammation can negatively impact the vagus nerve, leading to various health issues. Adding anti-inflammatory foods into your diet can support vagal tone and promote better health. Inflammation is often linked to chronic diseases like heart disease, diabetes, and autoimmune disorders. When inflammation is high, vagal tone tends to be low, compromising your body's ability to regulate stress and maintain balance. An anti-inflammatory diet helps counteract this, supporting your vagus nerve and overall wellness.

Including specific anti-inflammatory foods in your diet can make a significant difference. Omega-3-rich foods like salmon, flaxseeds, and walnuts reduce inflammation. Salmon is packed with EPA and DHA, types of omega-3 fatty acids that have a strong anti-inflammatory effect. Flaxseeds and walnuts provide alpha-linolenic acid (ALA), another form of omega-3 that supports heart health and reduces inflammation. Antioxidant-rich fruits such as berries and cherries are also beneficial. Blueberries, strawberries, and raspberries contain antioxidants that help fight oxidative stress and inflammation. Cherries contain anthocyanins, compounds that reduce inflammation and muscle pain, making them a great addition to your diet.

Vegetables like spinach and kale are nutritional gems that support overall health. Spinach is high in vitamins A, C, and K and magnesium, which helps reduce inflammation. Kale, known for its high antioxidant content, supports detoxification and inflammation reduction. Additionally, spices and herbs like turmeric and ginger are renowned for their anti-inflammatory properties. Turmeric contains curcumin, an ingredient with potent anti-inflammatory effects. Adding turmeric to your meals can aid in reducing inflammation and support joint health. Ginger, with its gingerol compounds, reduces inflammation and aids digestion, making it a great addition to your diet.

Adding these anti-inflammatory foods into your daily meals can be simple and delicious. Start your day with a smoothie packed with berries and flaxseeds. Blend a handful of blueberries, strawberries, and raspberries with a tablespoon of flaxseeds, some spinach, and almond milk for a nutritious breakfast. For lunch, enjoy a kale and quinoa salad topped with walnuts. Toss fresh kale with cooked quinoa, add some cherry tomatoes, cucumbers, and a handful of walnuts, then drizzle with olive oil and lemon. Dinner can feature grilled salmon with steamed spinach and turmeric rice. Season the salmon with lemon and herbs, grill it to perfection, and serve with a side of spinach sautéed in olive oil and garlic. Season your rice with a pinch of turmeric for added flavor and anti-inflammatory benefits.

For snacks, keep it simple yet nutritious. A mix of cherries and almonds makes for a delicious and anti-inflammatory snack. Cherries provide antioxidants, while almonds offer healthy fats and protein. By adding these ingredients to your meals, you can enjoy a mix of flavors while supporting your vagus nerve and overall health.

To help you get started, here are some sample meal plans and recipes:

- For **breakfast**, blend a berry and flaxseed smoothie. Combine a handful of mixed berries, a tablespoon of flaxseeds, a cup of spinach, and almond milk.
- For **lunch**, prepare a kale and quinoa salad with walnuts. Mix cooked quinoa with fresh kale, cherry tomatoes, cucumbers, and walnuts, then drizzle with olive oil and lemon juice.
- **Dinner** can be grilled salmon with steamed spinach and turmeric rice. Season the salmon with lemon and herbs, grill it, and serve with sautéed spinach and turmeric-infused rice.
- For a **snack**, enjoy a mix of cherries and almonds. These meals are delicious and support your vagus nerve.

GUT-BRAIN AXIS: FOODS THAT PROMOTE VAGAL TONE

The gut-brain axis, a critical link between the digestive system and the brain, plays a significant role in overall health. This two-way communication allows signals to flow from the gut to the brain and vice versa. At the core of this connection is the vagus nerve, which acts as a vital communication pathway. It not only regulates digestion but also influences mood and mental health. A healthy gut sends beneficial signals to the brain, fostering overall well-being, while an unhealthy gut may contribute to challenges such as anxiety and depression. Prioritizing gut health can strengthen vagal tone and enhance both mental and physical health.

Certain foods are particularly beneficial for maintaining a healthy gut and promoting vagal tone. Probiotic-rich foods like yogurt, kefir, and sauerkraut are excellent choices. These foods contain healthy bacteria that help balance your gut microbiota, improving digestion and overall gut health. Yogurt and kefir, for example, are fermented dairy products rich in probiotics. Sauerkraut, made from fermented cabbage, also provides these beneficial bacteria. Adding these foods to your meals will contribute to a healthy gut environment.

Prebiotic-rich foods such as garlic, onions, and bananas are equally important. Prebiotics are types of fiber that benefit the healthy bacteria in your gut, helping them thrive. Garlic and onions contain inulin, a prebiotic fiber that assists the growth of good gut bacteria. Bananas, particularly when slightly green, are a great source of resistant starch, another type of prebiotic that supports gut health. Including these foods in your meals can help maintain a balanced gut microbiota.

High-fiber foods like oats, beans, and lentils are also beneficial. Fiber acts as a food source for your gut bacteria, promoting their growth and activity. Oats are versatile and nutritious, providing soluble and insoluble fiber. Beans and lentils are big sources of fiber and protein, making them a great addition to your diet. Consuming high-fiber foods regularly can help support digestive health and enhance vagal tone.

Fermented foods like kimchi, miso, and kombucha offer additional benefits. Kimchi, a classic Korean dish made from fermented vegetables, is rich in probiotics and vitamins. Miso, a fermented soybean paste, is used in various dishes and provides beneficial bacteria. Kombucha, a fermented tea, is a refreshing beverage that supports gut health. Mixing these fermented foods into your diet can help maintain a healthy gut microbiota.

Adding these gut-friendly foods to your daily meals can be simple and delicious. Start your day with a bowl of Greek yogurt topped with banana slices and oats. Greek yogurt provides probiotics, while bananas and oats offer prebiotic fiber. For lunch, enjoy a hearty lentil soup with garlic and onions. This soup is not only flavorful but also packed with prebiotics and fiber. Dinner can feature stir-fried vegetables with miso sauce. Use a variety of colorful vegetables, add a spoonful of miso paste for flavor, and stir-fry until tender. For a snack, try sauerkraut and avocado on whole-grain toast. This combination provides probiotics, healthy fats, and fiber, making it a nutritious and satisfying option.

These foods can help create a healthy gut and enhance vagal tone. You can promote better digestion, mood, and mental health by focusing on probiotic-rich, prebiotic-rich, high-fiber, and fermented foods. Start with simple changes, like adding yogurt or kefir to your breakfast, including garlic and onions in savory dishes, snacking on bananas and nuts, or drinking kombucha as a refreshing beverage. These small tweaks to your diet can make a big difference in your overall well-being.

IMPORTANCE OF HYDRATION: STAYING WELL-HYDRATED

Staying hydrated is important for sustaining overall health and optimal vagus nerve function. Water is vital in all bodily functions, from regulating temperature to aiding digestion. When you stay well-hydrated, your body can efficiently transport nutrients, remove waste, and maintain cellular health. Proper hydration also supports blood circulation and keeps your skin healthy. This is particularly important for the vagus nerve, which thrives in a well-hydrated environment. When you're dehydrated, your body struggles to maintain balance, which can negatively impact vagal tone.

The connection between hydration and vagal tone is significant. Hydration ensures that the electrical signals responsible for controlling various bodily functions, including those managed by the vagus nerve, are transmitted smoothly. When your body is dehydrated, these signals can become erratic, leading to decreased vagal tone. This can make it harder for your body to manage stress, regulate digestion, and maintain a calm state. Staying well-hydrated helps maintain a stable environment for your vagus nerve, enhancing its ability to function effectively and supporting your overall health.

To maintain proper hydration, aim to drink about 15.5 cups (3.7 liters) of fluids daily for men and 11.5 cups (2.7 liters) for women. These guidelines are from the Mayo Clinic and include all fluids consumed, not just water. Your hydration needs vary based on activity level, climate, and overall health. If you're physically active, you'll need more water to replace fluids lost through sweat. Similarly, hot and humid climates increase your body's need for hydration. Pay attention to your body's signals and adjust your fluid intake accordingly.

Staying well-hydrated doesn't have to be complicated. Simple habits can make a big difference. Carry a water bottle with you throughout the day to ensure easy access to water. Setting water break reminders on your phone or using hydration apps can also help you remember to drink water regularly. Drinking a glass of water before each meal is another effective strategy. This helps with hydration, aids digestion, and prevents overeating. Adding flavor to your water with lemon or cucumber slices can make it more enjoyable and encourage you to drink more.

Hydrating foods are another excellent way to maintain fluid balance. Water-rich fruits like watermelon and strawberries are refreshing and contribute to your overall hydration. Watermelon is about 92% water, making it an excellent hydrating snack.

Strawberries are also rich in water and antioxidants, supporting hydration and overall health. Hydrating vegetables like cucumber and celery are great additions to your meals. Cucumbers are about 95% water and are low in calories, making them a perfect hydrating snack. Celery, with its high water content and fiber, helps keep you hydrated and supports digestion. Soups and broths are also effective hydrating meals. They provide essential nutrients and fluids, making them a great addition to your diet, especially in colder months.

Engaging in these strategies can help you stay well-hydrated and support your vagus nerve function. Carrying a water bottle, setting reminders, drinking water before meals, and adding flavorful ingredients to your water are simple yet effective ways to ensure adequate hydration. Including water-heavy fruits and vegetables in your diet can further enhance your hydration efforts. Remember, being well-hydrated is not just about drinking water; it's about maintaining a balance that supports all your bodily functions.

LIFESTYLE HABITS: DAILY ROUTINES FOR OPTIMAL HEALTH

The habits you cultivate profoundly impact your vagus nerve health. Lifestyle choices directly influence your vagal tone, which in turn affects your physical, mental, and emotional health. Participating in regular physical activity, maintaining adequate sleep, managing stress, and nurturing social connections are all essential components of a healthy lifestyle. These habits support your vagus nerve and improve your resilience, mood, and overall quality of life.

A Consistent physical routine is a cornerstone of a healthy lifestyle. Activities like walking, yoga, and swimming can significantly enhance vagal tone. Walking is a simple yet effective way to stay active. It improves cardiovascular health, supports weight management, and boosts mood. Yoga, combined with physical postures, breathing exercises, and meditation, is particularly beneficial for the vagus nerve. It promotes relaxation, reduces stress, and enhances flexibility.

Swimming is a low-impact exercise that is also a full-body workout, enhancing muscle strength, boosting cardiovascular health, and encouraging relaxation. Including activities like swimming in your routine can support healthy vagal tone and contribute to overall wellness.

Adequate sleep is another critical factor in supporting vagus nerve health. Maintaining a consistent sleep schedule helps regulate your body's internal clock, promoting better sleep quality. Aim for 7-9 hours of sleep each night. Consider activities such as reading, enjoying a warm bath, or practicing deep breathing techniques to unwind before bed. Minimize screen time and avoid stimulating activities for at least an hour prior to sleeping. Prioritizing rest helps support a healthy vagus nerve, which is key to your stress management.

Managing stress is essential for a healthy vagal tone. Techniques such as mindfulness and meditation are powerful tools in this process. Mindfulness encourages present-moment awareness without judgment. These exercises can be done during everyday activities like eating, walking, or washing dishes. Meditation, however, involves setting aside time to focus your mind and reach a state of deep relaxation. Additional practices like deep breathing, progressive muscle relaxation, and guided imagery can further reduce stress and support vagal tone.

Social relationships play a significant role in supporting vagus nerve health. Engaging in meaningful relationships and community involvement can enhance your emotional well-being and vagal tone. Make time for social interactions with friends and family. Participate in community activities, join clubs, or volunteer for

CHAPTER 10

causes you care about. These connections provide emotional support, reduce feelings of loneliness, and promote a sense of belonging. Strong social ties can buffer against stress, enhance happiness, and improve overall health.

Adopting and maintaining these healthy lifestyle habits can be straightforward with a few practical tips. Set aside specific times for daily exercise, such as a morning walk or an evening yoga session. Build a consistent sleep schedule by going to bed and waking up at the same time each day. Try to nurture a relaxing bedtime routine that includes calming activities and avoids screens. Practice mindfulness during daily tasks by focusing on the present moment and engaging your senses. Make time for social interactions by scheduling regular catch-ups with friends, participating in group activities, or joining community events.

Adding these lifestyle habits into your daily routine can support your vagus nerve health. Simple changes like regular exercise, consistent sleep, stress management, and nurturing social connections can significantly affect your physical, mental, and emotional health.

CHAPTER 11
REAL-LIFE CASE STUDIES

OVERCOME ANXIETY: SARAH'S JOURNEY

Imagine a bustling café where Sarah, a dedicated nurse, was constantly on edge. Balancing long shifts, family responsibilities, and personal obligations left her feeling overwhelmed. The weight of her anxiety was evident in every aspect of her life. She struggled to focus at work, her patience wore thin at home, and her social life dwindled as she withdrew from friends. Sarah's once vibrant personality seemed lost under the heavy cloud of chronic anxiety that had become her constant companion.

Sarah's journey towards discovering vagus nerve exercises began with a casual conversation with a colleague. The colleague noticed Sarah's distress and recommended she explore vagus nerve exercises. Initially skeptical, Sarah hesitated. She had tried various methods to manage her anxiety, from medication to traditional therapy, with limited success. However, the persistent encouragement from her colleague, coupled with her own curiosity, led Sarah to start researching. She spent evenings reading articles and watching videos about the vagus nerve and its potential benefits for anxiety relief.

Her research revealed several exercises designed to stimulate the vagus nerve. Sarah decided to start with diaphragmatic breathing, a technique she could easily incorporate into her daily routine. Before the day's chaos began each morning, she dedicated ten minutes to deep breathing. Sitting comfortably, she placed one hand on her chest and the other on her abdomen, focusing on slow, deep breaths that made her abdomen rise and fall. This simple practice helped her start the day with a sense of calm and control.

In addition to diaphragmatic breathing, Sarah integrated mindfulness meditation into her mornings. She found a quiet corner in her home, free from distractions, where she could sit and focus on her breath. In each session, she gently redirected her mind back to her breathing whenever it wandered. This practice not only reduced her anxiety but also improved her ability to stay present and engaged throughout the day. The combination of these two exercises became a cornerstone of her morning routine.

As she grew more comfortable with these practices, Sarah incorporated cold showers into her routine. Starting with her usual warm shower, she gradually reduced the temperature until she could stand under cold water for a few minutes. The initial shock of the cold water was challenging, but she quickly noticed the stimulating effects. The cold showers left her feeling refreshed and energized, providing a natural boost to her mood and resilience.

The results of these practices were profound. Over time, Sarah noticed a surprising reduction in her anxiety symptoms. She felt more relaxed and in control, even in high-pressure situations at work. Her focus and productivity improved, allowing her to perform her duties with greater efficiency and confidence. The sense of calm she cultivated through her morning routine carried over into her interactions with colleagues and patients, enhancing her professional relationships.

At home, the changes were equally remarkable. Sarah's enhanced emotional resilience allowed her to reconnect with her family and friends. She found joy in social interactions that she had previously dreaded. Her relationships deepened as she became more present and attentive, able to offer genuine support and empathy to her loved ones. The transformation in her mental health was evident to everyone around her, inspiring several friends and family members to explore vagus nerve exercises themselves.

Sarah's journey illustrates the transformative power of simple, consistent practices. By dedicating a few minutes each day to diaphragmatic breathing, mindfulness meditation, and cold showers, she was able to reclaim her life from the grip of anxiety. Her story is a testament to the potential of vagus nerve exercises to bring about profound improvements in mental health and overall well-being.

CHRONIC PAIN RELIEF: JOHN'S SUCCESS STORY

John worked as a construction manager, a job that demanded long hours on his feet and strenuous physical activity. Despite his strong physique, years of heavy lifting and repetitive motions took a toll on his body. He experienced chronic pain in his lower back and shoulders, making even simple tasks excruciating. The pain seeped into every aspect of his life, affecting his sleep, mood, and overall quality of life. John found himself avoiding activities he once enjoyed, and his relationships began to strain under the weight of his constant discomfort.

A turning point came when John visited a physical therapist. The therapist suggested he explore vagus nerve exercises as a complementary approach to his treatment plan. Initially skeptical, John had tried various pain relief methods with little success. However, his curiosity was piqued, and he began researching the potential benefits of vagus nerve stimulation. He read articles, watched videos, and gradually became convinced it was worth trying. The idea of using the body's natural mechanisms to relieve pain intrigued him, and he decided to give it a shot.

John started with gentle yoga poses, incorporating them into a daily stretching routine. Each morning, he dedicated time to practicing poses that focused on relieving tension in his back and shoulders. Poses like Cat-Cow and Child's Pose became staples in his routine. He found that these gentle movements helped to stretch and relax the muscles around his spine, providing immediate relief. The consistent practice of yoga not only alleviated his pain but also improved his flexibility and mobility over time. He felt a renewed sense of control over his body, which had been missing for years.

John introduced body scan meditation into his evening routine to further enhance his relaxation. Before bed, he would lie down in a quiet room each night and guide his attention through his body, starting from his toes and moving up to his head. This practice allowed him to identify and release areas of tension, promoting a deep sense of relaxation. The body scan meditation became a powerful tool for managing his pain and improving his sleep quality. As his body relaxed, his mind followed, providing a peaceful end to his day.

John also experimented with cold exposure therapy, adding weekly ice baths to his regimen. He started with cold showers, gradually building his tolerance before transitioning to full ice baths. Initially, the cold shocked his system, but he soon began to appreciate the stimulating effects. The ice baths significantly reduced his inflammation and muscle soreness, accelerating his recovery from physical exertion. He noticed that his pain levels decreased after each session, and his overall energy levels improved.

CHAPTER 11

The results of these practices were transformative. John experienced a significant reduction in his chronic pain, allowing him to return to activities he had long avoided. His increased mobility and flexibility made daily tasks easier and more enjoyable. The combination of yoga, meditation, and cold exposure therapy not only alleviated his physical discomfort but also enhanced his mental health. He felt more energized, slept better, and found a new sense of balance in his life. John's success story underscores the power of vagus nerve exercises in managing chronic pain and improving overall quality of life.

IMPROVED DIGESTION: EMILY'S TRANSFORMATION

In a bustling city, Emily worked as a marketing executive. Her days were packed with back-to-back meetings, tight deadlines, and constant stress. Despite her professional success, Emily struggled with chronic digestive issues that seemed to overshadow her achievements. She often experienced severe bloating, discomfort, and irregular bowel movements, which made her daily life challenging. These issues left her feeling drained and affected her mood and overall energy levels.

A turning point came when Emily sought advice from a nutritionist. The nutritionist, concerned about Emily's well-being, recommended she explore vagus nerve exercises to help manage her digestive problems. Initially, Emily was skeptical. She had tried various diets and supplements with little success. However, her curiosity got the better of her, and she began researching the benefits of vagus nerve stimulation. She discovered a wealth of information that piqued her interest and decided to try it.

Emily started with diaphragmatic breathing before and after meals. She found a quiet spot in her home, sat comfortably, and placed one hand on her chest and the other on her abdomen. Focusing on slow, deep breaths, she ensured her stomach rose and fell with each breath. This simple practice helped her relax and prepare her digestive system for food. It also aided digestion after meals, reducing the discomfort she usually felt. Over time, this routine became an integral part of her meal times.

In addition to diaphragmatic breathing, Emily made significant dietary changes. Following her nutritionist's advice, she incorporated probiotic-rich foods into her daily diet. She started eating yogurt and kefir for breakfast, added sauerkraut and kimchi to her lunch and dinner, and snacked on probiotic supplements. These changes helped balance her gut microbiome, promoting healthier digestion and reducing bloating. Emily also ensured her diet was rich in prebiotic foods like garlic, onions, and bananas, further supporting her gut health.

Emily also introduced gentle abdominal massages into her routine. Each morning and evening, she would spend a few minutes gently massaging her abdomen in a circular motion. This practice stimulated her digestive organs and promoted bowel movements, enhancing her overall digestive function. The massages became a soothing ritual that helped her start and end her day positively.

The results of these practices were remarkable. Emily experienced a significant reduction in bloating and discomfort, which had previously been a constant source of distress. Her digestion became more regular, and she no longer struggled with the irregular bowel movements that had plagued her for years. These improvements in her digestive health had a ripple effect on her overall health. She noticed a boost in her mood and energy levels, which made her more productive and focused at work. Her social life also improved, as she no longer had to worry about digestive issues interfering with her plans.

Emily's transformation highlights the power of vagus nerve exercises in improving digestive health. By incorporating diaphragmatic breathing, dietary changes, and abdominal massages into her daily routine, she was able to reclaim her life from the grip of chronic digestive problems. Her story is an inspiring example of how simple, consistent practices can lead to profound improvements.

ENHANCED EMOTIONAL HEALTH: MICHAEL'S EXPERIENCE

Michael, a high-powered attorney, often found himself grappling with intense emotional swings. His demanding job required long hours and high-stakes decision-making, leaving him mentally and emotionally drained. Michael's emotional regulation issues ranged from sudden outbursts of anger to overwhelming feelings of sadness. These mood swings affected his relationships both at work and at home, creating a cycle of stress and isolation. He felt trapped, unable to break free from the emotional turmoil that clouded his life.

It was during a particularly challenging period that Michael's psychologist suggested he explore vagus nerve exercises. Initially, Michael was skeptical. He had tried various forms of therapy and medication, but none provided lasting relief. However, his curiosity led him to research the vagus nerve and its impact on emotional health. He read articles and watched videos, intrigued by the potential benefits. The idea of using simple exercises to stimulate his vagus nerve and improve his emotional well-being seemed worth exploring.

Michael began with loving-kindness meditation, a practice recommended by his psychologist. Each morning, he set aside time to sit in a quiet space, close his eyes, and focus on generating feelings of compassion and kindness. He started by directing these feelings towards himself, then gradually extended them to loved ones, acquaintances, and even people he struggled with. This daily practice helped him develop a sense of emotional resilience and stability. The act of cultivating positive emotions had a profound effect on his mood, making him feel more balanced and at peace.

In addition to loving-kindness meditation, Michael incorporated resonant frequency breathing into stressful situations. Whenever he felt overwhelmed or on the verge of an emotional outburst, he practiced breathing at a steady rhythm of five to six breaths per minute. This technique helped synchronize his heart rate with his breath, promoting a state of calm. The immediate effect of resonant frequency breathing allowed him to navigate stressful moments with greater ease and composure. It became a reliable tool for managing his emotions in real time.

Recognizing the importance of social connections for emotional health, Michael also made a conscious effort to engage in regular community involvement. He joined local clubs and volunteered for community projects, activities that allowed him to connect with others and build meaningful relationships. These social engagements provided a sense of belonging and support. The positive interactions and shared experiences helped him feel more grounded and less isolated.

The changes Michael experienced were significant. His emotional resilience and stability improved, allowing him to handle stress and challenges more effectively. The mood swings that once dominated his life became less frequent and less intense. His relationships benefited immensely from his newfound emotional balance. At work, colleagues noticed his improved demeanor and ability to stay calm under pressure. At home, his interactions with family members became more positive and supportive. Michael's overall happiness and life satisfaction increased, making him feel more fulfilled and content.

Michael's experience underscores the transformative potential of vagus nerve exercises for emotional well-being. By integrating

CHAPTER 11

loving-kindness meditation, resonant frequency breathing, and social engagement into his routine, he was able to reclaim control over his emotions and improve his quality of life. His story is a powerful example of how simple, consistent practices can lead to profound mental and emotional health improvements.

These real-life case studies illustrate the diverse benefits of vagus nerve exercises, from reducing anxiety and chronic pain to improving digestion. Each story highlights these simple practices' profound impact on their quality of life.

CHAPTER 12
INTEGRATING VAGUS NERVE EXERCISES INTO DAILY LIFE

MORNING ROUTINES: STARTING YOUR DAY RIGHT

The way you start your morning can significantly impact your entire day. A structured morning routine with vagus nerve exercises can reduce stress and anxiety, preparing your body and mind for the challenges ahead. Dedicating a few minutes each morning to these exercises can enhance your mental and physical health. Imagine beginning your day with a sense of calm and readiness rather than stress and rush.

A detailed morning routine can make all the difference. Start with diaphragmatic breathing for 5-10 minutes upon waking. This involves sitting or lying comfortably, placing one hand on your chest and the other on your abdomen. Breathe deeply through your nose, ensuring your abdomen rises more than your chest, then exhale slowly through your mouth. This simple practice activates your parasympathetic nervous system, reducing anxiety and promoting relaxation.

Next, engage in gentle stretching or yoga for 10-15 minutes. This could include poses like Child's Pose, Cat-Cow, or gentle spinal twists. Stretching awakens your body and stimulates the vagus nerve. Follow this with 5-10 minutes of mindfulness meditation. Find a quiet spot, sit comfortably, and focus on your breath. Allow thoughts to come and go without any judgment, bringing your attention back to your breath each time your mind wanders. This practice can clear your mind and enhance mental clarity for the day ahead.

Finish your routine with a cold shower or a splash of cold water on your face for 1-2 minutes. The cold exposure triggers the mammalian diving reflex, stimulating the vagus nerve and boosting alertness. If a cold shower feels too daunting, start with just your face or the back of your neck. Over time, you may find yourself more comfortable with longer durations.

Maintaining consistency is essential for experiencing the advantages of this routine. Establish a regular wake-up time to help normalize your body's internal clock. Prepare the night before by laying out your yoga mat and setting up a quiet space for meditation. Use alarms or reminders to ensure you don't skip your routine. The more regular your practice, the more ingrained it will become in your daily life.

Adding these simple practices into your morning can set a positive tone for the day. The benefits extend beyond reducing stress and anxiety; they enhance your overall well-being, making you feel more balanced and prepared for whatever comes your way.

MIDDAY PRACTICES: STAYING BALANCED

As the day progresses, it's natural to experience a dip in energy and an increase in stress. This midday slump can hamper your focus and productivity, making it harder to stay balanced. Incorporating vagus nerve exercises into your midday routine can counteract this fatigue, helping you manage stress and maintain energy levels.

CHAPTER 12

Taking a few moments to care for your nervous system can improve your performance for the rest of the day.

One effective way to integrate vagus nerve exercises is through deep breathing exercises. During your lunch break, find a quiet spot to sit comfortably. Spend 5-10 minutes practicing deep breathing. Sit with your back straight, close your eyes, and take slow, deep breaths through your nose. Focus on making your exhales longer than your inhales, which encourages vagal activation.

This practice calms your mind and helps reset your body's stress response, preparing you for the afternoon ahead. Physical activity also plays a big part in maintaining midday balance. Consider taking a short walk or gentle physical activity for 10-15 minutes. This could be a brisk walk around the block, light stretching, or even a few yoga poses.

Movement stimulates the vagus nerve and refreshes your body, improving circulation and boosting your energy levels. Plus, stepping away from your desk and getting some fresh air can clear your mind and enhance your focus.

Mindfulness or body scan meditation can further reset your mind during the day. Find a quiet spot to sit or lie down without interruptions. Spend 5-10 minutes focusing on each part of your body, starting from your toes and working your way up to your head. Become aware of any areas of tension and consciously release them. This practice helps you become more aware of your physical state and promotes relaxation, reducing midday stress and improving your mental clarity.

Staying hydrated is another simple but effective way to support your vagus nerve health. Set a reminder to drink a glass of water during your midday break. Proper hydration supports overall bodily functions and enhances your ability to manage stress.

Keeping a water bottle with you can be a good reminder to stay hydrated during the day.

Integrating these practices into a busy schedule might seem challenging, but with some planning, it becomes manageable. Use your lunch breaks effectively by setting aside specific times for these exercises. Set reminders on your phone or use apps designed to prompt you to take breaks and practice mindfulness. Find a quiet space at work or home where you can perform these exercises without disruption. Even a few minutes of dedicated practice can significantly impact your overall well-being.

Consider the experience of Lisa, a project manager who struggled with afternoon fatigue and stress. By incorporating deep breathing and short walks into her midday routine, she noticed a significant reduction in her afternoon slump. Her focus improved, and she felt more energized and productive. Similarly, a graphic designer, Tom, found that adding mindfulness meditation during his lunch break helped him manage stress and maintain a balanced state throughout the day.

These midday practices offer practical tools to help you stay balanced and energized. By dedicating a few moments to your routine, you can counteract stress and fatigue, enhancing your focus and productivity for the rest of the day.

EVENING ROUTINES: PREPARING FOR RESTFUL SLEEP

Imagine you're winding down after a long day. The evening is the perfect time to engage in practices that prepare your body and mind for restful sleep. Evening vagus nerve exercises can help reduce evening stress and anxiety, helping you unwind and improve sleep quality. By dedicating time in the evening to these exercises, you create a soothing transition from the day's activities to a peaceful night's rest.

Start your evening routine with gentle stretching or yoga for 10-15 minutes. This helps release the tension that builds up throughout the day. Poses like Seated Forward Bend, Child's Pose, or Legs-Up-the-Wall are excellent choices. These gentle stretches relax your muscles and stimulate the vagus nerve, creating a state of calm and readiness for sleep.

Follow this with 5-10 minutes of diaphragmatic breathing to calm your mind. Find a comfortable position by sitting or lying down, then rest one hand on your chest and the other on your abdomen. Focus on inhaling and exhaling slowly and deeply. This method of breathing engages the parasympathetic nervous system, lowering stress levels and getting your mind ready for relaxation.

Next, engage in guided imagery or body scan meditation for 10-15 minutes. Find a quiet space, close your eyes, and visualize a peaceful scene or focus on each part of your body from head to toe, releasing tension as you go. This practice helps you detach from the day's stresses and promotes deep relaxation, making it easier to fall asleep and stay asleep through the night.

Avoid screens and stimulating activities before bed to further support your evening routine. The blue light cast by screens can interfere with your body's natural sleep-wake rhythm, making it more difficult to fall asleep. Instead, engage in calming activities like reading a book, listening to soothing music, or taking a warm bath.

Consistency is key to making your evening routine a regular habit. Set a consistent bedtime to regulate your body's internal clock. Establish a calming atmosphere for sleep by ensuring your bedroom is cool, dim, and peaceful. Using calming scents like lavender can also enhance the relaxation process. Think about utilizing a diffuser with lavender essential oil or putting a sachet of dried lavender beneath your pillow. These small changes can significantly improve your sleep quality over time.

Consider the story of Emma, a busy nurse who struggled with insomnia for years. By incorporating an evening routine of gentle stretching, diaphragmatic breathing, and guided imagery, she experienced a significant improvement in her sleep quality. Emma found that she fell asleep faster and stayed asleep longer, waking up feeling more refreshed and energized.

By dedicating time each evening to these simple yet effective practices, you can create a peaceful transition from the day's activities to a restful night's sleep.

OVERCOMING BARRIERS: CONSISTENCY AND COMMITMENT

Maintaining a regular practice of vagus nerve exercises can be challenging. Many people face obstacles that make it difficult to stay consistent. One common barrier is a lack of time. Busy schedules can leave little to no room for self-care, making it easy to skip exercises. Initial skepticism or lack of motivation can also hinder progress. It's hard to commit when you're not convinced of the benefits. Additionally, establishing new habits can be difficult, especially if you're already juggling multiple responsibilities. Distractions and interruptions from work, family, or technology can further disrupt your practice.

To overcome these barriers, start by setting realistic goals and starting small. Instead of aiming for an hour-long session, begin with five minutes and gradually increase the duration as you become more comfortable. This approach makes the practice feel more manageable and less daunting. Finding accountability partners or joining support groups can also provide motivation and

CHAPTER 12

encouragement. Sharing your progress with others or participating in group sessions can make the experience more engaging and less isolating.

Using habit-tracking tools and apps can help you stay on track. There are numerous apps designed to remind you of your exercises and track your progress over time. Visualizing your progress can be a good motivator, reinforcing your commitment to the practice. Creating a dedicated space for your exercises can also enhance consistency. Whether it's a corner of your room or a spot in your garden, having a specific place for your practice can make it easier to focus and minimize distractions.

Consistency is needed for achieving and maintaining the benefits of vagus nerve exercises. Regular practice leads to gradual improvement in vagal tone, supporting sustained mental and physical health benefits. Over time, you'll notice enhanced emotional resilience, reduced anxiety, and improved overall well-being. These long-term benefits are a powerful incentive to stick with your routine.

By addressing these common barriers and implementing practical strategies, you can maintain a consistent practice and reap the long-term benefits of vagus nerve exercises. It's about finding what works for you, setting small, achievable goals, and staying committed to your progress. The journey may have its challenges, but with persistence and dedication, you'll experience profound improvements in your mental and physical health.

CONCLUSION

As we come to the end of this journey together, it's clear that the vagus nerve holds remarkable importance in both mental and physical health. This nerve, running from the brainstem through the neck and down to the abdomen, is responsible for activating the parasympathetic nervous system. It helps our bodies achieve homeostasis, promoting relaxation, reducing inflammation, and enhancing overall well-being. Understanding and stimulating the vagus nerve can lead to profound benefits in how we manage stress, pain, trauma, and even our digestive health.

Throughout this book, we've explored a variety of exercises designed to stimulate the vagus nerve. From deep diaphragmatic breathing and mindfulness meditation to cold exposure and gentle yoga, these practices are accessible and easy to add to your daily life.

Now, it's your turn to take action. Begin by incorporating a few simple exercises into your daily routine. Start with deep breathing or a short mindfulness session each morning. Slowly add more exercises as you become comfortable. Keep track of your progress and note the changes in your physical and mental health.

CONCLUSION

Remember, consistency is key. The benefits of these exercises build up over time, leading to lasting improvements. Community and social connections also play a big role in enhancing vagal tone and overall health.

As you embark on this road towards improved health, remember that small, consistent steps can lead to profound transformation. The exercises and techniques outlined in this book are about addressing specific health issues and nurturing a balanced, resilient, and vibrant life. By committing to regular practice, you are investing in yourself and unlocking the potential for a healthier, happier you.

In the words of one of our success stories, "It's not just about the exercises—it's about creating a life where you feel in control and at peace." Embrace the power of the vagus nerve and let it guide you toward a future filled with calm, balance, and vitality. Your journey to better health starts now.

REFERENCES

1 StatPearls. (n.d.). *Neuroanatomy, cranial nerve 10 (vagus nerve).* Retrieved from https://www.ncbi.nlm.nih.gov/books/NBK537171/

2 Cleveland Clinic. (n.d.). *Vagus nerve: What it is, function, location & conditions.* Retrieved from https://my.clevelandclinic.org/health/body/22279-vagus-nerve

3 Unyte. (n.d.). *Dr. Stephen Porges' Polyvagal Theory.* Retrieved from https://integratedlistening.com/polyvagal-theory/

4 National Center for Biotechnology Information. (2022). *Clinical perspectives on vagus nerve stimulation. PMC.* Retrieved from https://www.ncbi.nlm.nih.gov/pmc/articles/PMC9093220/

5 PubMed. (n.d.). *The vagus nerve and the inflammatory reflex.* Retrieved from https://pubmed.ncbi.nlm.nih.gov/23169440/

6 National Center for Biotechnology Information. (2017). *Vagus nerve stimulation modulates complexity of heart. PMC.* Retrieved from https://www.ncbi.nlm.nih.gov/pmc/articles/PMC5682746/

REFERENCES

7 Frontiers in Aging Neuroscience. (2023). *Neuroimmunomodulation of vagus nerve stimulation and aging.* Retrieved from https://www.frontiersin.org/journals/aging-neuroscience/articles/10.3389/fnagi.2023.1173987/full

8 PubMed. (2022). *Vagus nerve stimulation: An update on a novel treatment.* Retrieved from https://pubmed.ncbi.nlm.nih.gov/35158102/

9 National Center for Biotechnology Information. (2011). *The polyvagal theory: New insights into adaptive reactions.* PMC. Retrieved from https://www.ncbi.nlm.nih.gov/pmc/articles/PMC3108032/

10 Cleveland Clinic. (n.d.). *Fight anxiety with a strong vagus nerve.* Retrieved from https://health.clevelandclinic.org/what-does-the-vagus-nerve-do/

11 National Center for Biotechnology Information. (2022). *A comprehensive review of vagus nerve stimulation for epilepsy.* PMC. Retrieved from https://www.ncbi.nlm.nih.gov/pmc/articles/PMC8898319/

12 National Center for Biotechnology Information. (2023). *Humming (Simple Bhramari Pranayama) as a stress buster.* PMC. Retrieved from https://www.ncbi.nlm.nih.gov/pmc/articles/PMC10182780/

13 National Center for Biotechnology Information. (2022). *Role of vagus nerve stimulation in the treatment of depression.* PMC. Retrieved from https://www.ncbi.nlm.nih.gov/pmc/articles/PMC10614462/

14 Morningside Acupuncture NYC. (n.d.). *Acupuncture and the vagus nerve.* Retrieved from https://www.morningsideacupuncturenyc.com/blog/acupuncture-and-the-vagus-nerve

15 Parsley Health. (n.d.). *8 vagus nerve stimulation exercises that help you relax.* Retrieved from https://www.parsleyhealth.com/blog/how-to-stimulate-vagus-nerve-exercises/

REFERENCES

16 National Center for Biotechnology Information. (2018). *Breath of life: The respiratory vagal stimulation model*. PMC. Retrieved from https://www.ncbi.nlm.nih.gov/pmc/articles/PMC6189422/

17 Medical News Today. (n.d.). *4-7-8 breathing: How it works, benefits, and uses*. Retrieved from https://www.medicalnewstoday.com/articles/324417

18 National Center for Biotechnology Information. (2013). *Assessment of the effects of pranayama/alternate nostril breathing*. PMC. Retrieved from https://www.ncbi.nlm.nih.gov/pmc/articles/PMC3681046/

19 National Center for Biotechnology Information. (2022). *Effect of resonance breathing on heart rate variability*. PMC. Retrieved from https://www.ncbi.nlm.nih.gov/pmc/articles/PMC8924557/

20 National Center for Biotechnology Information. (2022). *Transcutaneous vagus nerve stimulation could improve cognition*. PMC. Retrieved from https://www.ncbi.nlm.nih.gov/pmc/articles/PMC9599790/

21 Frontiers in Integrative Neuroscience. (2022). *Polyvagal theory: A science of safety*. Retrieved from https://www.frontiersin.org/journals/integrative-neuroscience/articles/10.3389/fnint.2022.871227/full

22 Healthline. (n.d.). *8 breathing exercises for sleep: Techniques that work*. Retrieved from https://www.healthline.com/health/breathing-exercises-for-sleep

23 YogaUOnline. (n.d.). *Yoga for better sleep: 5 restful restorative poses*. Retrieved from https://yogauonline.com/yoga-practice-teaching-tips/yoga-practice-tips/yoga-for-better-sleep-5-restful-restorative-poses/

24 Institute for Functional Medicine. (n.d.). *Understanding PTSD*

REFERENCES

from a polyvagal perspective. Retrieved from https://www.ifm.org/news-insights/understanding-ptsd-from-a-polyvagal-perspective/

25 Verywell Mind. (n.d.). *Grounding techniques for coping with PTSD and anxiety.* Retrieved from https://www.verywellmind.com/grounding-techniques-for-ptsd-2797300

26 Parsley Health. (n.d.). *8 vagus nerve stimulation exercises that help you relax.* Retrieved from https://www.parsleyhealth.com/blog/how-to-stimulate-vagus-nerve-exercises/

27 Trauma Healing. (n.d.). *Somatic experiencing: Supporting trauma resolution and recovery.* Retrieved from https://traumahealing.org/

28 National Center for Biotechnology Information. (2020). *Mindful eating: A review of how the stress-digestion axis influences eating behavior.* PMC. Retrieved from https://www.ncbi.nlm.nih.gov/pmc/articles/PMC7219460/

29 Confidence in Eating. (n.d.). *How mindful breathing can help you with emotional eating.* Retrieved from https://confidenceineating.com/mindful-breathing-emotional-eating/

30 Charlie Health. (n.d.). *5 vagus nerve exercises to help you chill out.* Retrieved from https://www.charliehealth.com/post/vagus-nerve-exercises

31 National Center for Biotechnology Information. (2016). *Role of the vagus nerve in the development and treatment of diseases.* PMC. Retrieved from https://www.ncbi.nlm.nih.gov/pmc/articles/PMC5063945/

32 Nourish Therapeutic Yoga. (n.d.). *Yoga for the vagus nerve.* Retrieved from https://www.nourishtherapeuticyoga.com/blogs/news/yoga-for-the-vagus-nerve

33 Healthline. (n.d.). *Sun salutation sequences A, B, and C: A complete*

REFERENCES

guide. Retrieved from https://www.healthline.com/health/fitness/sun-salutation-sequence

34 YogaUOnline. (n.d.). *6 vagus nerve exercises to boost well-being*. Retrieved from https://yogauonline.com/yoga-practice-teaching-tips/yoga-practice-tips/6-ways-to-stimulate-your-vagus-nerve-with-yoga-and-breathing/

35 Spanish Yoga Retreat. (n.d.). *Vagus nerve yoga: A practical guide for health and happiness*. Retrieved from https://spanishyogaretreat.com/vagus-nerve-yoga/

36 National Center for Biotechnology Information. (2021). *The effects of mindfulness and meditation on vagally mediated health outcomes. PMC.* Retrieved from https://www.ncbi.nlm.nih.gov/pmc/articles/PMC8243562/

37 National Center for Biotechnology Information. (2019). *Mindfulness, interoception, and the body: A contemporary review. PMC.* Retrieved from https://www.ncbi.nlm.nih.gov/pmc/articles/PMC6753170/

38 National Center for Biotechnology Information. (2011). *Loving-kindness and compassion meditation: Potential for health benefits. PMC.* Retrieved from https://www.ncbi.nlm.nih.gov/pmc/articles/PMC3176989/

39 National Center for Biotechnology Information. (2018). *Nature-based guided imagery as an intervention for state anxiety. PMC.* Retrieved from https://www.ncbi.nlm.nih.gov/pmc/articles/PMC6176042/

40 National Center for Biotechnology Information. (2019). *Effects of cold stimulation on cardiac-vagal activation in humans. PMC.* Retrieved from https://www.ncbi.nlm.nih.gov/pmc/articles/PMC6334714/

41 Mayo Clinic Health System. (n.d.). *Cold-water plunging health*

REFERENCES

benefits. Retrieved from https://www.mayoclinichealthsystem.org/hometown-health/speaking-of-health/cold-plunge-after-workouts

42 National Center for Biotechnology Information. (2021). *Use of cryotherapy for managing chronic pain*. PMC. Retrieved from https://www.ncbi.nlm.nih.gov/pmc/articles/PMC8119547/

43 Healthline. (n.d.). *Wim Hof breathing: Method, benefits, and more*. Retrieved from https://www.healthline.com/health/wim-hof-method

44 National Center for Biotechnology Information. (2016). *Anti-inflammatory properties of the vagus nerve*. PMC. Retrieved from https://www.ncbi.nlm.nih.gov/pmc/articles/PMC5063949/

45 National Center for Biotechnology Information. (2022). *Vagus nerve and underlying impact on the gut microbiota*. PMC. Retrieved from https://www.ncbi.nlm.nih.gov/pmc/articles/PMC9656367/

46 Mayo Clinic. (n.d.). *Water: How much should you drink every day?*. Retrieved from https://www.mayoclinic.org/healthy-lifestyle/nutrition-and-healthy-eating/in-depth/water/art-20044256

47 Neurodivergent Insights. (n.d.). *Improve vagal tone*. Retrieved from https://neurodivergentinsights.com/blog/how-to-improve-vagal-tone

48 Verywell Mind. (n.d.). *How vagus nerve exercises saved my mental health*. Retrieved from https://www.verywellmind.com/vagus-nerve-exercises-saved-my-mental-health-7096204

49 Isha Health. (n.d.). *Exploring vagus nerve stimulation: A potential path for anxiety relief*. Retrieved from https://www.isha.health/post/exploring-vagus-nerve-stimulation-a-potential-path-for-anxiety-relief

50 National Center for Biotechnology Information. (2022). *Vagus

REFERENCES

nerve stimulation: A personalized therapeutic approach. PMC. Retrieved from https://www.ncbi.nlm.nih.gov/pmc/articles/PMC9776705/

www.ingramcontent.com/pod-product-compliance
Lightning Source LLC
Chambersburg PA
CBHW031155020426
42333CB00013B/680